www.htional.com

Bringing you products from all Harcourt Health Sciences companies including Baillière Tindall, Churchill Livingstone, Mosby and W.B. Saunders

- ▷ **Browse** for latest information on new books, journals and electronic products

- ▷ **Search** for information on over 20 000 published titles with full product information including tables of contents and sample chapters

- ▷ **Keep up to date** with our extensive publishing programme in your field by registering with eAlert or requesting postal updates

- ▷ **Secure online ordering** with prompt delivery, as well as full contact details to order by phone, fax or post

- ▷ **News** of special features and promotions

If you are based in the following countries, please visit the country-specific site to receive full details of product availability and local ordering information

USA: www.harcourthealth.com

Canada: www.harcourtcanada.com

Australia: www.harcourt.com.au

⚜ Baillière Tindall   ◿ CHURCHILL LIVINGSTONE   Ⓜ Mosby   🅦 W.B. SAUNDERS

The Theory and Practice of
Therapeutic Touch

*We are not discovering reality,
but participating in its creation.*
MICHAEL TALBOT

For Churchill Livingstone:

Publishing Manager: Inta Ozols
Project Development Manager: Katrina Mather
Designer: George Ajayi

The Theory and Practice of
Therapeutic Touch

Jean Sayre-Adams RN RPTT MA
Director, The Sacred Space Foundation, Cumbria, UK

Stephen G Wright RN RCNT DipN Dans MSc RPTT FRCN MBE
Associate Professor, St Martin's College, Lancaster, UK; Chair, The Sacred Space Foundation, Cumbria, UK

with contributions by

Francis C Biley PhD MSc (Manchester) BNurs (Wales) RMN RGN PGCE FETCert
Lecturer in Nursing Studies, University of Wales College of Medicine; Co-ordinator, International Region of the Society of Rogerian Scholars

Michael Richardson RN BN (Hons)
Staff Nurse, Infectious Diseases Unit, University Hospital of Wales, Cardiff, UK

SECOND EDITION

CHURCHILL
LIVINGSTONE

EDINBURGH LONDON NEW YORK PHILADELPHIA
ST LOUIS SYDNEY TORONTO 2001

© Longman Group Limited 1995
© Harcourt Publishers Limited 2001
© Photographic artwork John Houlihan

CHURCHILL LIVINGSTONE
An imprint of Harcourt Publishers Limited

📖 is a registered trademark of Harcourt Publishers Limited

The right of Jean Sayre-Adams and Stephen G Wright to be identified
as authors of this work has been asserted by them in accordance with
the Copyright, Designs and Patents Act 1988

First published 1995
Second edition 2001

ISBN 0 443 0708 22

British Library Cataloguing in Publication Data
A catalogue record for this book is available from the British Library

Library of Congress Cataloging in Publication Data
A catalog record for this book is available from the Library of
Congress

Note
Medical knowledge is constantly changing. As new information
becomes available, changes in treatment, procedures, equipment and
the use of drugs become necessary. The authors and the publishers
have taken care to ensure that the information given in this text is
accurate and up to date. However, readers are strongly advised to
confirm that the information, especially with regard to drug usage,
complies with the latest legislation and standards of practice.

The
publisher's
policy is to use
**paper manufactured
from sustainable forests**

Printed in China

Contents

Preface

If you don't know what to do,
Just put your hands on them and love them
Pannatier

When words fail, there can be no better way to convey to another that 'I care' than by touch. However, there are many ways of touching, and even more ways in which others might respond. In the modern world of high-tech medicine and drugs, complex professional roles, attempts at cost control and higher through-put, people can often become more distant from, rather than closer to, those who seek to heal them.

It cannot be coincidence that, worldwide, millions of people have turned to complementary therapists for help. If these therapies have witnessed a growth boom in recent years, there has been an equally strong backlash. Sceptics, traditionalists, religious fundamentalists and many others have conducted a rearguard action to hold back the tide. Yet demands for access to complementary therapies escalate inexorably, perhaps because they offer an intimacy of contact that is lacking in many aspects of health care. The complementary therapies all tend to focus on a close helping relationship between therapist and patient, and they offer comfort and sometimes healing when other measures have failed or are no longer appropriate. The complementary therapies also tend to focus on the individual, seeking to help the whole person and the many aspects of wellbeing, not just the disease process. For some, they may even offer a spiritual dimension that could be lacking in their lives. Complementary therapies, compared to many other health care techniques, are usually pleasant to experience and pain free – they are often used in conjunction with meditation, relaxation, music, guided imagery and so on. Thus the focus may frequently be on putting people in the best condition for self-healing to occur, rather than relying upon complex technical interventions.

Many of the therapies also place a heavy reliance upon touch, but what sort of touch? How does ordinary touch differ from that which is therapeutic? What is the difference between the touch used when washing someone's skin or helping them to move, and that which seeks to help and heal? Can such therapies work *with* conventional medicine or do they go against the grain?

One technique, Therapeutic Touch (TT), has been gaining increased attention in recent years. As discussed in Chapter 1, we have reservations about even including TT as a complementary therapy. To us it is a core quality relevant to all healing and health care practices.

TT relies upon the belief that people are not just solid matter to which our everyday perceptions are accustomed; we do not end at our skin. As we discuss in Chapters 1 and 2, other perceptions of human beings are available to us – as consciousness, energy and so on. Through appropriate training, it is possible for us to become aware of this, and for each of us to tap into that awareness. Thus we can work with this new knowledge and participate in the healing of others – indeed, in this different world view 'self' and 'other' merge. When this book was first published in 1995, we used Rogers' theory of Unitary Human Beings to underpin our approach to TT. As a model to understand what may be happening in TT, it still provides us with a useful approach and is helpful to beginners in providing a structure for learning the theory and practice of TT. However, as we discuss at several points in the book, describing such models as Rogers' as useful is all that is needed. Anyone who has deepened their knowledge and practice in TT learns that no model, no theory, is adequate to describe what is taking place. There are so many unknowns and mysteries that may one day be discovered. On the other hand, perhaps being mysterious, as with many other approaches to healing, is part of what makes it 'work'.

It is possible, through the practice of TT, to help and heal another by holding the context in which relaxation and maximum health can occur. The TT practitioner does not simply transfer healing energy to another, but participates in a highly intricate and complex process, with the intention of putting the person in the best position for self-healing to take place.

TT does not require people to reject established health care techniques, rather it seeks to work with them in a complementary and supportive way, and indeed we may come to see in time that it is central to any healing and health care work.

Many health care workers find themselves ideally placed to incorporate TT into their everyday practice, as the many examples in this text will illustrate. It is relatively easy to learn, requires no special equipment or drugs and costs little more than the practitioner's time. It seems to help many people while also being safe – the worst that can happen is nothing at all.

We have compiled this book in response to the growing demand for more information. It will explore the background, research, practice and education of TT. We are grateful to all the contributors who have given much time and effort to this project – enabling us to produce what will be a guide for those who seek to develop the practice of TT themselves. Through the work of the Sacred Space Foundation, a charity dedicated to the teaching and development of TT in the UK, many thousands of health care workers and others have now learned of the benefits of TT, both for themselves and others. TT opens a gateway into healing that is available to all of us. We hope this book will provide you with the insights and opportunities, and incentive, to take a step through and journey along the healing path for yourself.

Jean Sayre-Adams and Steve Wright
Cumbria

Authors' note

As TT is relevant to a wide range of those who work in healing and health care, we have sought to make our ideas relevant to all, while drawing upon our nursing background and the leading work done on TT in nursing. Throughout the text, for simplicity, when we have referred to nurses this is in the generic sense and includes midwives and health visitors. Carers and other health care workers practising TT need only change the word 'nurse' to their own preferred title. Again, for simplicity, we have used the word 'patient' when referring to someone 'receiving' TT, although this is done with some reservations, as outlined in Chapter 1.

Acknowledgements

We are grateful to Janet Venn, Carol Horrigan, Ann Mills, Jill Fawke and Barbro Perkins for providing material used as case studies in parts of the text. Felicity Rankin, whose story appears on page 92 drew the picture on the back cover.

1

An introduction and background to Therapeutic Touch

Jean Sayre-Adams   Steve Wright

Recent thinking on the nature of energy
Concepts of human energy
The emergence of Therapeutic Touch
The challenge of scepticism
A theoretical background
Why us?

■ *The real voyage of discovery consists not in seeking new lands but in seeing with new eyes.*

MARCEL PROUST

Therapeutic Touch (TT) is a modern version of one of the oldest of therapies – the use of touch as a means of comfort and healing. At the same time the understanding of why it has lasted down through the centuries is at the cutting edge of many modern scientific disciplines, quantum physics for example.

This chapter will give a general overview of TT, which traces some of the history of the laying on of hands. Although Chapter 2 will explore the research on TT, some historical background is also included to offer some additional dimensions.

Evidence of the use of touch as a method of healing can be traced back 15 000 years to drawings found on the walls of caves. Early Eastern philosophical and religious literature, Greek mythology, ancient Egyptian artefacts, native American myths, all contain some mention of touch as a means used to heal. Evidence for the use of laying on of hands to heal human illness in ancient Egypt is found in the Ebers Papyrus dated 1552 BC. Four centuries before Christ, the Greeks used touch therapy in their Asklepian temples for healing the sick. The writings of Aristophanes detail the use of laying on of hands in Athens to restore a blind man's sight and return fertility to a barren woman. Hippocrates (460–377 BC) recorded, 'It has often appeared, while I have been soothing my patients that there was a singular property in my hands to pull and draw away from the affected parts, aches and diverse impurities by laying my hand upon the place and by extending my fingers toward it' (cited in MacManaway & Turcan 1983).

The Bible has many references to laying on of hands for both medical and spiritual applications (see Chapter 2). Healing was considered as much part of the early Christian ministry as preaching or administering the sacraments. In some European countries, members of royal families were thought to heal with the 'royal touch'. This belief lasted until the reign of William IV and, some would argue, was continued in the life and work of the already near-legendary Princess Diana. Many of these earlier attempts at healing were based upon a belief in the power of Jesus, the king or a particular healer. Even now, many healers act in the name of a spirit guide, particular guru (dead or alive) or believing they have a special dispensation from God. In Europe from the fifteenth to the nineteenth century, doctors and occultists such as Paracelsus and Fludd, and healers such as Mesmer, theorised about the likely magnetic nature of 'energies' instead of believing that they were tapping into 'powers' belonging to others.

Touching as a part of the healing act was widely used by both shamans and traditional practitioners until the rise of Puritan culture in Western Europe during the 1600s. At that time too, there was a shift away from what came to be seen as 'primitive' healing to modern scientific medicine (Baldwin 1986, Jahnke 1985). Achterberg (1990) writes that:

> *Puritan culture equated touch with sex, which was associated with original sin. Religious and scientific views, which rejected traditional practices, gave succour to a movement that sought to exterminate those who persisted in using them. Millions of people, especially women, acting as healers were caught up in general persecutions and exterminations of those involved in practices which were little understood and often drawn within the same net as witchcraft.*

Because of the rise of scientific medicine and the strong puritanical ethic, all unnecessary touch was discouraged. It was not until the 1950s that touch as a therapeutic intervention began to be researched (Dossey 1988).

All cultures have developed their own customs and taboos around touching. It has been suggested that British/American culture is one of the most touch-deprived in the world. Jourard (1964) watched pairs of people engaged in coffee shops in Puerto Rico, Paris, Florida and London. He counted the number of times one person touched another during one hour. In Puerto Rico the average was 180, in Paris 110, but in Florida it was only 2 and London 0.

It is important to note here that not all patients, because of their cultural upbringing, want to be touched or feel comfortable in being touched by all people. Therefore, before any kind of touching is initiated with patients it is necessary to take into consideration the social context and cultural differences concerning touch. For example, there may be differences relating to different parts of the body that it is considered acceptable to touch. Touch that is acceptable between two women may be inappropriate when offered between men and women. Similarly, levels of acceptable touch between men may also differ. Additional dimensions are brought in through religious and other cultural effects. It is usually inappropriate for a Muslim woman to receive hands-on nursing from a male nurse, and so on.

At the same time, everyone needs touch. Infants cannot survive without it, and studies show that the need for touch does not diminish as people grow older. Indeed, older people may suffer most acutely from lack of touch because of separation from, or loss of, family and friends. They are also affected by various social stigmas and expectations of how older people should behave, such as assumptions that they should no longer need or desire close physical contact (Marr & Kershaw 1998). Yet touch also functions as an effective communication channel for the older person at a time of life when other forms of communication may be less acute (Baldwin 1986).

Touch is probably one of the most highly used senses. The skin is the largest sense organ of the body, and touch is the first sense to develop in the human embryo, the one most vital for survival. Much of the infant's first information about the world is gained from the way he or she is touched during the birthing process, and touch continues to be used to learn about our environment. It is through the skin that knowledge about the external world is communicated to the brain, and in turn people convey to others information about themselves. A piece of skin the size of a small coin such as a penny or a quarter contains more than 3 million cells, 12 feet of nerves, 100 sweat glands, 50 nerve endings and 3 feet of blood vessels. It is estimated that there are about 50 receptors over 100 square centimetres, a total of about 900 000 sensory receptors per person (Montague & Matson 1979).

Touching has always been an integral part of the work of health care, but it is the way we touch that determines whether it will be an act of healing or a mechanistic procedural act. Many health care professionals move forward intuitively to hold a hand or to touch an arm as a gesture of reassurance. Hand holding has been described as a positive means of communication and one that seems to break down barriers (Knable 1981). Through the mechanism of touch, one can convey feelings of caring and understanding to the patient (Schmahl 1964). Other feelings, intentionally or unintentionally, can also be conveyed. For example, judgemental attitudes are revealed in the way we do or do not touch patients. It is very important that health care professionals first examine their own feelings about the meaning of touch before using it as a therapeutic tool.

In order for any kind of touch to be truly effective it must be given authentically by a warm, genuine, caring individual to one who is willing to receive it. Touch cannot and should not be packaged and dispensed. Insincere or inappropriate touching may be more upsetting to the patient than none at all.

Recent thinking on the nature of energy

Quantum physics is just one of the new disciplines that is beginning to explore some of the complex energy relationships between people and their environment. There has been a paradigm (a map or blue-print of reality) shift from the older mechanical world view of the Newtonian pragmatists to the new perspective of an interconnected holistic universe as envisioned by post-Einsteinian thinkers. Newtonian physics is mechanistic and reductionist – it views the person as essentially a group of body systems interacting in predictable ways. Post-Einsteinian thinking encourages a more holistic view of people – not just an interrelationship of body organs, but connected with and part of the 'energy' or pattern of the whole universe. Modern physicists see the universe as a dynamic web of interrelated events, none of which functions in isolation (Capra 1976).

At this point, however, a note of caution needs to be considered, having used the word 'energy'. First of all, modern science currently recognises only four forms of energy – gravitational, electromagnetic, and strong and weak nuclear (Dossey 1997). Something happens in healing work and in the practice of TT – people feel or experience things, changes in their state of health and wellbeing can be observed. Yet it is with some caution that this can be attributed to 'energy' – a word now much used and abused in descriptions of healing, especially in much 'new age' commentary. The ineffable nature of healing may lead us to attribute results or experiences to a particular 'something' in our search for description and certainty.

That 'something' may happen in the practice of TT there is no doubt, as the research and case studies cited in this text confirm.

However, it may be presumptuous to conclude that this is a result of 'energy'. It may be that some form of subtle energy that has yet to be identified is at work but, until this is found to be the case, practitioners of TT need to be cautious in how the word is used. To do otherwise exposes approaches to healing such as TT and its practitioners to ridicule or scepticism – neither of which do much to encourage understanding or the furthering of knowledge or research. Those who work with TT may find their understanding of healing alters radically, and their experience may be fascinating as their knowledge and skills deepen. It may be that they witness, and the patient experiences, a subtle form of energy at work. It may be that this energy is just another way that known energies are operating that we do not yet quite understand. It may also be that something else is taking place, so that senses of 'energy' and other experiences are merely projections of an underlying process that is much more intricate and complex (or perhaps very simple).

Bohm (1973) wrote of quantum theory as follows:

...there has been too little emphasis on what is, in our view, the most fundamentally different new feature of all, i.e. the intimate interconnectedness of different systems that are not in spatial contact, and later ... the parts are seen to be in immediate connection, in which their dynamical relationships depend, in an irreducible way, on the state of the whole system (and indeed on that broader system in which they are contained, extending ultimately and in principle to the entire universe). Thus one is led to a new notion of unbroken wholeness which denies the classical idea of analysability of the world into separately and independently existent parts.

In simpler language, this new physics believes that energy and mass are the same thing, every living thing in the universe is a pattern of moving energy, and that all living beings are interconnected to all other living things and interacting with them all the time. These ideas require nurses, other health care workers and all who work with TT to move from the concrete to the abstract, because almost everything we have been taught about the nature of the universe and reality is challenged. Our belief systems can determine our view of reality. For example, some beliefs about the world see it as a planet orbiting the sun, others as riding on the back of a turtle (native Americans), others as flat. Similarly, traditional thinking on the nature of the body as taught in many nursing and medical schools relies heavily on the solid and predictable behaviour of atoms, molecules and cells. A quantum physics view reveals a very different universe of enormous interchange of energy – the body not so much a solid fixed mass, but in constant movement of energy internally and externally.

Concepts of human energy

Concepts of essential life energy go by a variety of names in different disciplines and different parts of the world. However, scholars who have made a study of these energies have found strong correlation among all of them. Three major perspectives on vital energies that have significantly influenced recent Western thought are Indian, Chinese and Egyptian. Krieger (1975) chose the Indian philosophy as a framework in which to do her pioneering work with TT.

From the perspective of this philosophy, TT is primarily concerned with the use of prana, which is difficult to translate and define in Western culture, but may be seen simply as the vigour and vitality of the body and all the underlying processes, such as growth, breathing and healing. In a healthy individual, prana is abundant, while a lack of prana is the corollary of disease. Chakras are also part of this framework. They can be thought of in Western terms as energy transformers, which take in subtle energy and distribute it to the major glands, nerve centres and organs of the body. Chakras are considered the centre of consciousness in this philosophy instead of the brain.

Some scientists in the Western world are moving away from the Newtonian understanding of life and illness. Instead of taking human beings apart to learn about them and why they become ill – identifying the component parts and how they operate or fail, and then how to fix them – they are moving towards the Einsteinian concept. Einstein was searching for a unified field that would embrace all time and space. The post-Einsteinian viewpoint of vibrational medicine sees the human being as a multi-dimensional organism made up of physical/cellular systems in dynamic interplay with complex regulatory energy fields. Vibrational medicine attempts to heal illness by manipulating these subtle energy fields by working with the energy of the body instead of manipulating the cells through drugs or surgery. Therefore, the perspective here is of consciousness being present in all the cells, not just as a product of brain activity. For example, each cell is seen as part of a 'river of consciousness' by Chopra (1989), a practising endocrinologist and former chief of staff of a major Massachusetts hospital.

Talbot (1991), in his book *The holographic universe*, suggests that consciousness is in the energy field of the person. Martha Rogers and her students (Malinski, Barnett, Parsey, Newman, Quinn, Cowling) are the cutting-edge nurse theorists whose ideas relate more to this post-Einsteinian concept, and it is these theorists that this book will explore (while not discounting those who place TT in an Eastern philosophical framework).

The emergence of Therapeutic Touch (TT)

Dr Dolores Krieger, then Professor of Nursing at New York University, became intrigued as she watched her friend Dora Kunz, then President of the US Theosophical Society, practice laying on of hands. Krieger went on to learn laying on of hands herself, practised it and researched it before beginning to teach it to her Master's degree students in a programme called 'Frontiers in Nursing' in the early 1970s. It was at this time that she coined the name Therapeutic Touch (TT) for this particular form of laying on of hands. Capital letters are used for the first letter of each word to distinguish it from other forms of touch that may have a therapeutic effect, including any kind of touching intervention such as massage, stroking or hand holding. Krieger's students went on to do good quality research on TT (see Chapter 2) and today it is mainstream nursing practice in the United States, largely due to these students, many of whom teach in major nursing schools and universities.

The 'mainstream' issue is important, for TT is often lumped with other therapies as a complementary therapy. A core underpinning of the approach to TT in this book is that it is not complementary to orthodox practice but core. TT is an approach to healing that can and should be an attribute of all those who work in health and healing, enhancing established approaches and enriching the potential for healing to emerge.

TT is now viewed as a natural human potential, which can be learned and practised by anyone who has the 'intention' to help or heal. This intention is at the core of the TT process and is described as an attempt to focus completely on the wellbeing of the patient in an act of unconditional love and compassion (Quinn & Strelkaukas 1993). For this reason TT has been called a 'healing meditation' (Krieger et al 1979). More detailed discussion of these aspects of TT takes place in Chapter 2.

In the beginning, Krieger and others took their framework for supporting TT from Eastern philosophic thought (indeed, similarities between Eastern and Western mysticism and quantum physics are noted by many mystics and scientists). However, since the 1970s, research has become more sophisticated as the branch of physics known as quantum mechanics has expanded. Along with this, scholars of Rogers have made the theory of Unitary Human Beings clearer and, for many, the framework for and definitions of TT have evolved closely with it. Thus two distinct frameworks in the development of TT are emerging. The first is that taken by Krieger and colleagues based on Eastern philosophy, the second is based on Rogers and quantum physics, and supported strongly by Quinn and other Rogerian scholars in their research (Society of Rogerian Scholars 1993).

Krieger's (1973) first definition of TT is, 'a derivative of laying on of hands that uses the hands to direct excess body energies from a person in the role of healer to another for the purpose of helping or healing that individual'. Two years later she added, 'although derived from the laying on of hands, it differs from it in that TT is not performed within a religious context. The person in the role of healer does the act of TT while in a meditative state and is motivated by an interest in the needs of the patient' (Krieger 1975).

Another definition, which came from the Nurse Healer's Professional Association (NHPA 1992), an association of nurses in the US who practise TT, is, 'a contemporary interpretation of several ancient healing practices, (TT) is a consciously directed process of energy exchange during which the practitioner uses the hands as a focus to facilitate healing'.

'HEALERS', 'HEALEES' AND HOLISM

We have already in this text slipped into traditional usage of words such as nurse or patient, and in TT circles the words healer and healee are frequently used. The idea of 'energy' exchange (or transfer) is often seen as a linear process from practitioner to client. The implied causality and the separation of the practitioner and client into two interacting human fields is too simplistic for many teachers and practitioners, and some theorists. This issue will be returned to in subsequent chapters. At this stage, it is useful to share a note of caution about creating separate roles for those involved in TT. Although we inevitably have to discuss TT in terms of roles of nurse and patient or practitioner and client, these may be seen only as stepping stones towards a deeper understanding of what TT is all about.

TT is much more intricate and complex than simple cause and effect. Furthermore a healer–healee relationship is not holistic, it is reductionist. Holism is about the oneness of all things, not separation into distinct roles. Healer–healee is just like doctor–patient – a dualistic separation of one from another that suggests one working with or doing to another. Whichever the case, despite the almost universal claims by those working in healing ways to holistic principles, to speak then of healer and healee is a contradiction in terms, a therapeutic oxymoron. It is not possible to assert that 'healers' work holistically, yet follow the old medical model of setting themselves apart from the one that comes to them for help.

A therapy is not necessarily holistic. Despite the claims of many enthusiasts about their particular therapy, be it orthodox or complementary, that they work in 'holistic ways', holistic practice is by no means guaranteed. It is just as easy to find complementary practitioners who are as obsessed with their particular technique as any mainstream practitioner might be with their own bit of health technology. What seems to be of significance in healing is not just the technique, but the quality of the relationship with the practitioner – relationships characterised by trust, mutuality, intention, openness, trust, compassion and love, i.e. 'right relationship'. Right relationship is a hallmark of holistic practice, and it is this that may be the trigger that sets off the inherent capacity of people to heal themselves (Wright & Sayre-Adams 2000).

Thus, certain approaches to healing may work regardless of techniques simply because the 'patient' believes in or has faith in the therapy and the practitioner, feels good in their presence and gets a relaxation response (a feature hitherto often dismissed as the placebo response). These alone may be sufficient to switch the patient into healing by boosting the autoimmune response (Pert 1997). Hippocrates commented that some people recover simply because of their satisfaction with the goodness of the doctor. Florence Nightingale famously described nursing as, 'putting the patient in the best condition for nature to act' (Nightingale 1869). In other words, something about the way we are with patients may be as significant, if not more so, than what we do. Being a healing presence, in a healing relationship with another, may be the most powerful force toward healing. Indeed, when we enter such healing relationships, notions like patient and doctor, healer and healee, self and other disappear. We may perceive, even for a brief moment, that mystical point when all once-firm barriers fall away and everything is present in the here and now; that sacred space where 'you' and 'me' simply slip into being part of all that is, and the healing moment is known.

Healing emerges from this space. This healing may or may not include curing, the resolution of a particular disease. Indeed it is quite possible to die and yet be healed. Healing, with its roots in the Anglo-Saxon 'haelan' meaning hale, whole, hearty, concerns our sense of wholeness, of being connected with the self and that which is beyond the self. An illness may be terminal, but a person may be healed because fear of death is lost, old hurts have been resolved, or he or she may come to see beyond the brief flash of worldly existence. Healing can mean simply 'feeling good about myself for the first time in ages' as one chronically ill 'patient' working with one of the authors has recently said. He went on to 'give up the drink' and get a job and renew many of his relationships. Technically speaking he is still a sick man and his physical illness is little changed. Yet he is different in the way he is now being in the world – more confident, more participative, more active, more whole.

Meanwhile, those who practice as healers and call themselves such, risk limiting the arguably wondrous force they are working with. Healing is core to health care, and part of every health care practitioner's work to some degree whether consciously so or not. Yet, aggravated by wariness of examining or even talking about healing (or simply using 'healing' interchangeably and confusingly with 'curing') in orthodox circles, notions of healing seem to have become colonised almost entirely by the complementary therapies movement. Healing itself is emerging as a separate therapy in its own right. This may be seen as a worrying trend if healing is deemed something that certain (nominated) healers do, while others get on with some other part of the patient's health care. Thus we may reach a situation of, 'I go to my doctor for this, my aromatherapist for that, my healer for …'. In other words, we end up with a mere extension of the reductionist medicine so prevalent now.

A more worrying trend is the claim put forward by some healers that *they* can relieve or heal injury and illness (often against the odds of medical prognosis) (Charman 2000). This is fuel to the fire for the sceptics, who dismiss the claims of the healers because no causal agent can be identified. Healers reinforce this division when they say that *they* are involved in a cause–effect relationship, between healer and healee, when *they* apply intention to heal and use the 'power of healing' as a therapeutic agent in its own right. Regardless of how this power is interpreted (light, love, energy, etc.), the tendency is for those who call themselves healers to see *themselves* as the channelers or guides or transmitters of this force in some way from, by or through *them* to another. We have used the italics here to emphasise the essential reductionist approach at work – not much different in fact from the much maligned orthodox medical model – 'me doctor: you patient' – separateness is not holism. In this model, only the 'therapy' has changed, the 'healer' is just as separate from the 'healee' as other labels of nurse or doctor or therapist and patient.

We can get caught in this trap regularly. People in their distress may seek someone out because they have heard that he or she is a 'healer'. When encountering someone suffering this is hardly the place and time to get into complex ontological debates about what is going on in healing. It may not be the appropriate time to say, 'Well, actually, I'm not really doing the healing because you see we are both … etc., etc …' It is necessary to work with the person where they are – their expectations and understanding, accepting given labels and roles (which may indeed be necessary to the patient's healing process). They may be explored appropriately in more depth later, when deepening the patients' awareness of what is taking place may be part of their ongoing healing. From this may come an empowering realisation that they can be a significant determinant of their own health as active participants in the healing process, not merely passive recipients, and reach for themselves for a moment an understanding of the wonder that is healing.

The important point is that those working in healing, while working with vernacular terminology, do not allow themselves to get caught up in a reductionist view or the arrogant, ego-driven posture that they somehow heal another. Quite simply, they do not, nor do they have any evidence that they do. Something happens. It may be down to some subtle energy that we have yet to properly research and identify. It may be the result of some as yet hidden bodily self-righting mechanism. It may be God at work. We simply cannot be sure – except by the certainty that faith and experience can bring, but these have yet to be adequately tested in any randomised controlled trial.

A healing response that we can witness may emerge, but its cause is essentially ephemeral. It is the stuff of involvement with the patient in the search for healing and the necessary entering of a place of (as yet) essential mystery. We simply do not yet have the tools or the evidence to exactly, incontrovertibly, say what it is that takes place (Feinstein & Horwitz 1997), although everyone working with healing probably has their own personal view – to do otherwise leads to the scoffing of the sceptics and the fooling of ourselves

What seems to be critical about healing work is the intention towards healing, the coming together of one or more person in search of healing (although work on non-local healing suggests that it is not even necessary for the persons to be in the same physical place together, see for example Benson 1996, Dossey 1993). Thus by focusing our attention on healing, we enter a different world of healing full of potential. This is not a passive world of praying for the best or laying on of hands, standing back and expecting God to do the rest. Nor is it a world of the healer conducting the healing orchestra. It is a world of mutuality, of participation, where what seems to count is that we join consciously in the process, reuniting in a deeper awareness of that whole of which we are a part.

Many of us working in the realms of health and healing are blessed with certain professional titles and roles. Attachments to these roles, their agendas, their ways of viewing the world, may not always be helpful, and this includes the increasing trend for healing to be seen as a separate therapy conducted by healers (Hodges & Scofield 1995). A patient with a back pain can see an orthopaedic surgeon and be told it's a disc problem, they can see a psychologist and be told it could be stress related, another therapist will say it's the product of pent-up emotions, someone else would see a blocked chakra, another a playing out of karma, another a wound from a past life ... and so on and so on. It's all down to whatever spectacles of a particular therapeutic model the practitioner is wearing. Illness is not just about suffering, but may have deeper purposes, which are obscured by the spectacles we use to view the patient. Indeed, we have to be cautious that what we see may be simply a reflection of our own image in the glass of our viewer. We can simply never be sure what the healing for another entails. Beyond cures and our natural human desire to see another well, we simply do not know the healing path of another, it is forever veiled to us, although sometimes the 'healer' may catch a glimpse when the veil is lifted. Some common features reported by TT practitioners are:

- A deep sense of humility by the practitioner, who tends to shun the label 'healer'.

- Recognition that they can describe only a small part of what takes place, and even then that words are inadequate.

- That they, along with the patient, are participating in something, of which they are a part, yet is also much greater than them.

- That they are not in control of it. It works with them, perhaps because they are consciously participating, but whether or not it would be 'better' without them is an unknown.

- There is a sense of inevitability, of fate about the work. The one seeking healing has come together with that person at the time that is somehow right for them.

- They are not attached to outcomes. They recognise their natural human desire to want someone to be well, but see this as something to set within a wider context. They do not pray or ask for a disease to be cured, but wish for the healing and wholeness of the other, whatever form that might take.

- They rest in their work without the need for certainty or absolutes.

- They are fairly 'well rounded' human beings – having worked on the healing of themselves, their ego attachments and so on to enable them to be more relaxed and available with another without their own 'stuff' (such as the desire for power) getting in the way.

- They are very conscious of the quality of relationships in the healing process.

We can all play around with our healing techniques, models of assessment, diagnostic tools and panoply of pills and potions. They work – to a degree – but may leave us as actors on the comic–tragic stage of those we see as others. How much more powerful is this healing work when we relax a little and let go of our fixed roles, agendas and blinkered vision. We can do our usual work by all means, but need to remember to find that place in ourselves where we can sit back and let it happen – in wonder.

The challenge of scepticism

An example of how some sceptics can manipulate views on TT to their own, perhaps dubious ends became well known in 1998. The *Journal of the American Medical Association* published a study carried out for a school project by a 12-year-old girl (Emily) debunking claims that TT is an effective treatment. Her premise was that TT therapists claimed to use their hands to manipulate a 'human energy field' – that

TT researchers say that people have an energy field that is detectable by therapists. Twenty-one 'TT therapists' (however, later in the paper Emily said they were, '… neighbors (sic) who were willing to help me with my science project' – how did Emily find twenty-one TT therapists among her neighbours?) were asked to put their hands through two holes in a partition. Emily then flipped a coin to decide whether to put her hand above the therapist's right or left hand and asked the therapist to identify which of their hands was closest to Emily's hovering unseen hand. The correct hand was identified in only 44% of the 280 blind trails. The study concluded that, 'the practitioners' failure to substantiate the therapy's most fundamental claim is unrefuted evidence that it is groundless and that further professional use is unjustified' (Rosa et al 1998).

Of course, for TT practitioners the study did not test any critical variables related to TT at all. The ability to sense the 'energy field' of another is simply not a requirement of a TT practitioner, although it may be a useful guide. Furthermore, when practitioners do begin to sense the 'energy field' of another the kinaesthetic sense (which is the sense that is being used with the hands) is only one of many senses that may be used. Hearing, seeing (clairvoyance) or intuiting may be other ways. The study was set up more as a parlour game (much of the design and requirements of the study were similar to one conceived earlier by the magician James Randi) with no centring or intentionality as part of the study (see Chapter 4). Emily had grown up in a household with parents who were avowed sceptics and who were activists in trying to debunk TT. Her neutrality in the study was therefore questionable. Many studies have indicated the 'experimenter bias' effect, in which the beliefs of the experimenter tend to be confirmed. Most interesting was why a journal with the reputation of the *Journal of the American Medical Association* would publish, without question, an article submitted by a lay family and one physician. In the ensuing public debate and extensive media attention it became clear that TT was getting caught up in the hostilities that occasionally arise from certain fundamentalist religions and some quarters of the medical establishment.

Continued interest in and expansion of the practice of TT has not been inhibited, although the incident gives a demonstration of how far some might go, with less than honourable agendas, to block anything that does not fit with their world view. A similar outburst very nearly destroyed the Bristol Cancer Help Centre a decade ago when a combination of media hype, flawed research and rearguard action from some of the medical establishment sought to undermine the groundbreaking work this centre had undertaken. These examples provide useful lessons for TT practitioners and others in ensuring they have high standards of practice, sound theoretical frameworks and reliable research to draw upon.

Another avenue of objection are some minority concerns that complementary or alternative therapies, or techniques based on Eastern philosophical thought, lead, 'to the destruction of the soul and spirit in Hell' and see all complementary therapies as based on anti-Christian religions that, 'may lead to occult involvement' (Gennis 1992). There are concerns that the practice of TT is a 'heathen' activity, based on fear of the person opening up to an outside force. They see the allowing of the mind to go blank (as sometimes suggested in meditation practices) as an invitation to invasion by demonic spirits (Malinski 1993).

Furthermore, because TT is still difficult to demonstrate (other than through experiential exercises) or to measure in orthodox scientific ways, it has even been rejected as a hoax. This text will explore these issues in the detailed discussions of many aspects of TT in subsequent chapters.

Some are sceptical for positive reasons; seeking knowledge and understanding to prevent wholesale acceptance of distorted or dangerous practices. Others are sceptical for the hell of it; determined from that deep fearful place in their psyches to quash anything that does not fit neatly with their particular world view.

The modern scientific medical paradigm demands a rationale for all health care practices and this trend is fuelled by government-sponsored bodies such as NICE in the UK (the National Institute for Clinical Excellence) and similar organisations in other countries, which have immense influence over what therapies can and cannot be available to patients. As Abbot (2000), in a helpful survey of the current evidence for healing from randomised clinical trials, points out, 'hard evidence of effectiveness is increasingly required for therapeutic interventions' and 'emphasising clinical efficacy and cost-effectiveness of service provision, is likely to increase the pressure on therapies such as healing to expand their evidence base, preferably through randomised controlled trials'. Monitoring the research base for a particular treatment, making a judgement on its effectiveness and then recommending whether it should or should not be used is, at one level, a sound and seductive approach. This is especially so when we have to account for the spending of public money and the protection of the public from charlatanism and quackery.

And charlatanism and quackery there is in abundance, thickly layered with added spreadings of irresponsibility and non-account-ability. Leafing through the pages of any new age journal, or come to that much of the main stream press, reveals a plethora of adverts to attend for or train in healing. There is little evidence that users and students of such services are properly and safely vetted beforehand, or effectively followed up afterwards. Anyone can call themselves a healer (despite the efforts of organisations such as the National Federation of Spiritual Healers to set standards of training and practice). Such limitations, added to sloppy conceptualising such as the random use of words like 'energy', make it difficult for individuals and organisations from different viewpoints to work together, and add strength to the arguments of the bigots and hostile sceptics. However, there are some hopeful signs. There is an increasing quantity of good quality research becoming available to support practices such as TT, and much collaborative work being undertaken nationally and internationally to integrate what were the once highly polarised orthodox and complementary perspectives, for example by the Foundation for Integrated Medicine in the UK (1997), various committees of the European Union and a congres-sional committee on complementary and alternative medicine in the United States.

A theoretical background

Many theorists and teachers prefer to bring TT into a theoretical framework, which provides a useful foundation for practice and research, and may help to explain the processes of TT. In this instance, the discipline of nursing has provided a helpful approach in the work of Martha Rogers. This, however, is not to devalue or discount the extremely valuable work that has been done from other perspectives, such as drawing upon Eastern philosophical thought and practices. Rogers' model, The Science of Unitary Human Beings, is the framework that has provided a foundation for many and is used in this text as a basis to further our understanding and teaching of TT. However, this must be balanced with noting the above reservations about the limitations of any one model or theory in the reality of TT and other healing practices.

Rogers defines people as irreducible, indivisible, multi-dimensional energy fields integral with the environmental energy field (Rogers 1990). Energy transfer and the limited notions of energy are too simplistic in relation to Rogers' model, and a full explanation of her theory is found in Chapter 3. It is important to note that while there is increasing support for the Rogerian premise of a 'human energy field', to date there have been no accurate reports of investigations that measure interaction between such individual human fields. 'The reality of such interaction therefore remains axiomatic' (Quinn 1989).

'Healing' is another word that is uncomfortable for many. Quinn (1992) states that:

> *Healing, the emergence of right relationship at, between and among all the levels of human being, is always accomplished by the one healing. No one and no thing can heal another human being (but themselves). All healing is creative emergence, new birth, the manifestation of the powerful inner longing, at every level, to be whole.*

Quinn believes that the role of the nurse and others who work towards healing is to remove barriers to the healing process, and much of this is found in the quality of the relationship in the 'sacred space' of healing (Wright & Sayre-Adams 2000). 'Being with' someone in right relationship may be the switch that triggers the potential of someone to heal themselves, to which Nightingale and Hippocrates, mentioned above, have alluded. More recently it has been postulated that the TT practitioner knowingly participates in the mutual human–environment process by shifting consciousness into a state that may be thought of as a 'healing meditation'. Many think that this facilitates repatterning of the patient's energy field through a process of resonance, rather than 'energy exchange or transfer' (Cowling 1990, Krieger et al 1979, Quinn 1992).

The definitions in the literature now begin to change. Meehan (1993), a student of Krieger and a researcher, teacher and practitioner of TT herself, redefined TT as 'a knowledgeable and purposive patterning of patient–environmental energy field process'. Here, the nurse or other health care practitioner, 'assumes a meditative form of awareness and uses her/his hands as a focus for the patterning of the mutual patient–environment energy field process'.

Malinski (1993) retains some of Meehan's wording when she defines TT as, 'a health patterning modality whereby nurse and client participate knowingly in the changing human–environmental field process'. As can be seen, much of the theorising and research into TT has come from a nursing perspective, but has now spread out to embrace health care workers from a wide variety of backgrounds.

Quinn clearly brings TT into a more accurate Rogerian perspective when she discusses the interconnectedness of all our lives. She sees our consciousness as not separate and apart but integral with all consciousness. With the intentional use of our own consciousness, we can move towards the repatterning and healing of ourselves and others. She believes that it is possible in the act of 'centring' (see Chapter 4) to shift one's consciousness. This in turn may provide a template of sorts upon which the patient may repattern and balance their energy field, which permits healing to take place.

Quinn (1992) writes, 'Using the metaphor of sound, the pattern, or vibration of the nurse's consciousness becomes a tuning fork, resonating at a healing frequency, while the client has the opportunity within the mutual person–environment process to tune, to resonate, to that frequency.' In other words, one person (or more, as we shall discuss), who works consciously towards healing for another enables the other to begin their own process of self-healing.

This way of looking at TT is also consistent with the modern physicists. Bentov (1977), a biochemical engineer, appears to share this view when he writes:

...the real reality ... the microreality, that which underlies our solid reality ... is a rapidly pulsating matrix of fields of energy, an interference pattern of waves filling the vast vacuum of our bodies and continuing beyond them in a more diluted fashion ... we may look at a disease as an out-of-tune behaviour ... when a strong harmonising rhythm is applied to it, the interference pattern of waves, may start beating in tune again.

Research to date has suggested that laying on of hands can increase the rate of wound healing in mice (Grad et al 1961), the rate of growth in plants (Grad 1963), the rate of activity of the enzyme trypsin (Smith 1972) and the level of human haemoglobin (Krieger 1972). Outcome studies to date indicate that it can increase human haemoglobin levels (Krieger 1974), induce physiologic relaxation (Krieger et al 1979), decrease anxiety (Gange & Toye 1994, Garrard 1995, Heidt 1981, Olson & Sneed 1995, Olson et al 1992, Olson et al 1997, Quinn 1989), relieve pain (Barrington 1994, Gordon et al 1998, Keller & Bzdek 1986, Meehan 1985), lower diastolic blood pressure (Quinn 1989), reduce stress in hospitalised children (Kramer 1990) and accelerate wound healing (Wirth 1990, 1993, Wirth et al 1994). Detailed discussion of this research is included in Chapter 2.

This research cannot be ignored and, of course, much more yet needs to be done. But many health care practitioners find themselves drawn to TT for a different reason ... simply, that it seems to work.

ONE NURSE'S STORY – HOW I CAME TO TT

It was 04.00 as I sat down with a hot beverage at the nurses' station to start my charting. My eyes drifted down the long, dark hall at the Cancer Research Institute at the University of California and stopped at the door out of which I had come 5 minutes before. I tried to form the words in my mind that I would put in the chart of Joan, the 33-year-old woman whom I had known as a patient with leukaemia for over a year. Joan had experienced two remissions but was now in the hospital with a liver abscess. She had been admitted almost 72 hours before, on my shift and, as in her admissions before, I was her primary nurse. I identified with Joan in her role as a mother and wife, and greatly admired her courage in the way she approached her physical disease with her use of meditation, yoga and other 'alternative' approaches in her quest towards healing. She had been a wise teacher, not only to me but to many other world expert oncologists. A good deal of my time had been spent with her for the last 8 hours (we worked 12-hour shifts), for in spite of every known trick or technique or medication known to modern science available in a University Teaching Hospital, Joan was still not only febrile (up to 40°C), but was in intense pain – tossing, turning, moaning on her bed, unable to fall into sleep. While searching my repertoire for some way in which I could relieve her pain and give her some comfort, I remembered a class in Therapeutic Touch I had taken a few months earlier. At the time I hadn't felt I could integrate the technique into my high-tech nursing. It had been interesting but I felt I couldn't do Therapeutic Touch as well as the others in the class and also was not sure how it matched with my concept of nursing. To tell the truth, I was a little in awe or afraid of the whole idea. But Dee's [Dolores Krieger's] words came back to me, 'Anyone can do TT, anyone can use TT to increase comfort and decrease anxiety'. Joan was beyond judging me, so I gave it a go. I did TT with Joan for the next 10 minutes.

She had fallen asleep and here I was now wondering how to put into words the complexities of the whole interaction. I put her chart aside and did routine charting on my other patients. And then, a half hour later, Joan's light went on. What could I possibly do for her that I hadn't already done, I thought as I walked the distance to her room. 'Could you change my wet bedding?' Joan said sleepily as I walked in. Joan had been sweating profusely, her temperature had broken and was now 38°C and her pain was completely gone. I was 'blown away'. The next day my clinical supervisor and I went through all her notes to find some other explanation – not only for Joan's pain relief but for the normalisation of her temperature. We did not find it but, over the rest of Joan's hospitalisation, TT administered either by me or her husband, to whom I taught TT, was used to keep her free of pain and her temperature acceptable (along with the appropriate medications which had not been working before).

I know there could be many explanations for what occurred, but none seem to fit with what happened that night. All I know is, it seemed to work. I was able to help someone in need.

Why us?

Caring is a central concept underpinning the work of many health care workers. Nurses, for example, make this the principal focus of their activity. One way of expressing caring is through what Benner (1984) has called 'presencing' – 'being with' (Wright 1992) the patient in such a way that the patient feels not only cared for, in terms of the practical things that are done to help, but also cared about and valued as a person. This means, for example, that nurses and others can put aside issues of personalities and behaviours of patients and recognise their value as human beings and seek genuinely and sincerely to help them. Campbell (1984) has described this as a form of 'moderated love', where the relationship is not physical or sexual, but filled with the loving commitment or intention to help and heal another person towards their own deeper healing (which may not be what the practitioner sees as their (the patient's) healing).

Through caring we are not only able to help sick people recover, we can also help them to feel better in themselves. Even with a patient who may be dying, where getting better is not possible, carers can help by promoting comfort, relaxation, a sense of wellbeing and acceptance.

People who are sick or 'dis-eased' are far more likely to heal, and heal more quickly, when they are helped to feel better about themselves (Kitson 1988, Pert 1997). As the following chapters will explore, TT is underpinned by the notions of intentionality (the focused willingness on the part of the healer to help the patient) and helping people to feel better. This puts the patients in a better position to mobilise their own healing potential more effectively.

Thus when people feel better, they are far more likely to find, for example, improvements in wound-healing, fewer risks of postoperative complications and so on. In this sense, it is possible to construct a strong case for the cost-effectiveness of TT. If nurses, doctors and other health care workers can bring TT into their everyday practice, there are several knock-on effects. Most immediately this concerns those we define as 'patients', improving their general level of wellbeing so that they may heal themselves, 'being with' people in the 'sacred space' of healing (Wright & Sayre-Adams 2000). Perhaps one of the challenges for future research into TT is to demonstrate its cost-effectiveness. Time spent helping people to feel better may have cost–benefits to the health care system if people get better more quickly as a result.

Another factor is the effect upon the staff themselves. As will be discussed in greater detail in Chapter 4, the relationship of the energy fields between practitioner and patient is neither linear nor unidirectional. Care staff derive benefit from TT as well – for example, in terms of general wellbeing and collegiate relationships. There are implications here not only for patient care, but also for the health of the organisation, staff relationships and effectiveness.

Health Services tend to be the biggest single employers in many societies. They consume huge amounts of resources, occupy thousands of people and affect millions of others. Imagine the implications if every one of us and our millions of colleagues in other disciplines was empowered with the healing potential of TT! Such power would not only affect the patient–practitioner relationship, not just the health care system, but could help transform society as a whole.

REFERENCES

Abbot N C 2000 Healing as a therapy for human disease: a systematic review. Journal of Alternative and Complementary Medicine 6(2):159–169

Achterberg J 1990 Woman as healer. Shambhala, Boston

Baldwin L 1986 The therapeutic use of touch with the elderly. Physical and Occupational Therapy in Geriatrics 4:45–50

Barrington R 1994 A naturalistic inquiry of postoperative pain after therapeutic touch. In: Gaut D A and Boykin A (eds) Caring as healing; renewal through hope. National League for Nursing, New York.

Bentov I 1977 Stalking the wild pendulum. Dutton, New York

Benner P 1984 From novice to expert. Addison Wesley, New York

Benson H 1996 Timeless healing. Schuster, New York

Bohm D 1973 Quantum theory as an indication of a new order in physics: implicate and explicate order in physical law. Foundation of Physics 3:139–168

Campbell A 1984 Moderated love. SPCK, Edinburgh

Capra F 1976 The tao of physics. Bantam, New York

Charman R A 2000 Placing healers, healees, and healing into a wider research context. Journal of Alternative and Complementary Medicine 6(2):177–180

Chopra D 1989 Quantum healing. Bantam, New York

Cowling R W 1990 A template for unitary pattern-based nursing practice. In: Barret EAM (ed) Visions of Rogers' science-based nursing. National League for Nursing, New York

Dossey B 1988 Holistic nursing: a handbook for practice. Aspen, Gaithersburg, Maryland

Dossey L 1993 Healing words. Harper, San Francisco

Dossey L 1997 The forces of healing; reflections of energy, consciousness and the beef stroganoff principle. Alternative Therapies in Health and Medicine 3(5):8–14

Feinstein A R and Horwitz R L 1997 Problems in the 'evidence' of evidence-based medicine. American Journal of Medicine 103:529–535

Foundation for Integrated Medicine 1997 Integrated healthcare. FIM, London.

Gagne D, Toye R 1994 The effects of Therapeutic Touch and relaxation therapy in reducing anxiety. Archives of Psychiatric Nursing 8(3):184–189

Garrard C T 1995 The effect of therapeutic touch on stress reduction and immune function on persons with AIDS. Dissertation Abstract International. University microfilm no. 9537117

Gennis F 1992 Alternative roads to hell? Nursing Standard 6(44):42–43

Gordon A, Merenstein J, D'Amico F, Hudgens D 1998 The effects of therapeutic touch on patients with osteoarthritis of the knee. The Journal of Family Practice 47(40):271–277

Grad B 1963 A telekinetic effect on plant growth. International Journal of Parapsychology 5:117–133

Grad B, Cadore R J, Paul G I 1961 An unorthodox method of treatment of wound healing in mice. International Journal of Parapsychology 3:5–24

Heidt P 1981 Effect of Therapeutic Touch on anxiety level of hospitalised patients. Nursing Research 30:32–37

Hodges R D, Scofield A M 1995 Is spiritual healing a valid and effective therapy? Journal of the Royal Society of Medicine 88:203–207

Jahnke R 1985 The body therapies. Journal of Holistic Nursing. Spring 7–14

Jourard J 1964 The transparent self: self disclosure and wellbeing. Van Nostrand, Princetown

Keller E, Bzdek V M 1986 Effects of Therapeutic Touch on tension headache pain. Nursing Research 35(2):101–106

Kitson A 1988 On the concept of nursing care. In: Fairbairn G, Fairbairn S (eds) Ethical issues in caring. Gower, Aldershot

Knable J 1981 Handholding: One means of transcending barriers of communication. Heart Lung 10:1106

Kramer N 1990 Comparison of Therapeutic Touch and casual touch in stress reduction of hospitalised children. Paediatric Nursing 16(5):483–485

Krieger D 1972 The response of in-vivo human haemoglobin to an active healing therapy by direct laying on of hands. Human Dimensions 1:12–15

Krieger D 1973 The relationship of touch, with intent to help or heal, to subjects' in-vivo haemoglobin values: a study in personalised interactions. Proceedings of the American Nurses Association 9th Nursing Research Conference, San Antonio, TX. March 21–23, pp 39–78

Krieger D 1974 Healing by the laying on of hands as a facilitator of bioenergetic change: the response of in-vivo human haemoglobin. Psychoenergetic Systems 1:121–129

Krieger D 1975 Therapeutic Touch: the imprimatur of nursing. American Journal of Nursing 75:784–787

Krieger D, Peper E, Ancoli S 1979 Physiologic indices of Therapeutic Touch. American Journal of Nursing 14:660–662

MacManaway B, Turcan J 1983 Healing. Thorsons, Wellingborough

Malinski V 1993 Therapeutic Touch: the view from Rogerian nursing science. Visions: The Journal of Rogerian Nursing Science 1(1):45–54

Marr J, Kershaw B 1998 Caring for older people. Arnold, London.

Meehan T C 1985 The effects of Therapeutic Touch on experience of acute pain in postoperative patients. Dissertation Abstract International 46 795B. University microfilm no. 8510765

Meehan T C 1993 Cited in Malinska V (ed) Therapeutic Touch: the view from Rogerian nursing science. Visions: The Journal of Rogerian Nursing Science 1(1):45–54

Montague A, Matson F 1979 The human connection. McGraw Hill, New York

Nightingale F 1869 (1980 ed) Notes on nursing, what it is and what it is not. Churchill Livingstone, Edinburgh

Nurse Healers Professional Association 1992 Summer Newsletter. NHPA, New York

Olson M, Sneed N, Bonadonna R, Ratcliff J, Dias J 1992 Therapeutic touch in post-hurricane Hugo stress. Journal of Holistic Nursing 10(2):120–136

Olson M, Sneed N 1995 Anxiety and therapeutic touch. Issues of mental health nursing 16:97–108

Olson M, Sneed M, LaVia M, Virella G, Bonadonna R, Michel Y 1997 Stress induced immunosuppression and therapeutic touch. Alternative Therapies in Health and Medicine 3(2):68–74

Pert C 1997 Molecules of emotion. Scribner, New York

Quinn J F 1984 Therapeutic Touch as energy exchange: testing the theory. Advances in Nursing Science 6(1):37–45

Quinn J 1989 Therapeutic Touch as energy exchange: replication and extension. Nursing Science Quarterly 2(2):79–87

Quinn J F 1992 Holding sacred space: the nurse as healing environment. Holistic Nursing Practice 6(4):26–35

Quinn J F, Strelkauskas A 1993 Psychoimmunologic effects of Therapeutic Touch on practitioners and recently bereaved recipients: a pilot study. Advanced Nursing Science 15(4):13–26

Rogers M 1990 Nursing: science of unitary, irreducible, human beings: update 1990. In: Barrett E (ed) Visions of Rogers' science based nursing. New York, National League for Nursing

Rosa L, Rosa E, Sarner L, Barret S 1998 A close look at therapeutic touch. Journal of American Medical Association 279(13):1005–1010

Schmahl C 1964 Ritualism in nursing practice. Nursing Forum 11:74

Smith J 1972 Paranormal effects on enzyme activity. Human Dimensions 1:12–15

Society of Rogerian Scholars 1993 Visions. Journal of Rogerian Nursing Science, Pensacola

Talbot M 1991 The holographic universe. Harper Collins, New York

Wirth D 1990 The effect of non-contact therapeutic touch on the healing rate of full thickness dermal wounds. Subtle Energies 1(1):1–20

Wirth D 1993 full thickness dermal wounds treated with non-contact Therapeutic Touch: a replication and extension. Complementary Therapies in Medicine 1(3):127–132

Wirth D, Barrett M, Eidelman W 1994 Non-contact therapeutic touch and wound epithelialisation; an extension of previous research. Complementary Therapies in Medicine 2:187–192

Wright SG 1992 My patient – my nurse: the practice of primary nursing. Scutari, Harrow.

Wright SG, Sayre-Adams J 2000 Sacred space – right relationship and spirituality in healthcare. Churchill Livingstone, Edinburgh

2
A review of the literature and research

From an original chapter by Michael Richardson, with additions by Jean Sayre-Adams and Steve Wright

■ *There is the danger that the phenomenon may, like the butterfly that is pinned down for closer inspection, be destroyed in the attempts to understand it.*

DR JANET QUINN

What is Therapeutic Touch?

The earliest reference in the literature to Therapeutic Touch (TT) states:

> *Therapeutic Touch ... consists of the simple placing of the hands for about 10 to 15 minutes on or close to the body of an ill person, by someone who intends to help or to heal that person.*
>
> *(Krieger 1975)*

It implies that a process occurs, whereby the nurse (the healer) directs attention using the hands to achieve a therapeutic effect for the patient (the healee).

Krieger (1975) added that the practice of TT is a, 'natural potential in physically healthy persons who are strongly motivated to help ill people'; most definitions of TT agree with this account (Meehan 1990a, Quinn 1992, Wright 1987).

Later definitions by Krieger and other writers put emphasis on describing TT as an exercise in which the healer, intentionally through a process of meditation, acts as a channel for an assumed 'universal life energy', which actualises a healing process in the healee (Krieger et al 1979, Macrae 1988). For this reason TT has also been described as a 'healing meditation' (Peper & Ancoli 1976), and the underlying dynamic by which it has an effect is an exchange of this assumed energy (Quinn 1984).

A basic assumption of TT is that the interplay of energy accelerates a natural self-healing mechanism in the client, as the following description implies:

> *The transfer of energy from the person playing the role of healer is most usually little more than a booster until the patient's own recuperative system takes over. At best the healer accelerates the healing process.*
>
> *(Krieger 1979)*

It has been postulated that physical contact is not needed to perform TT because the treatment is based on the assumption that all living things are surrounded by an energy field that can be balanced using the hands (Carruthers 1992). The nature of this theorised energy field has not been empirically defined as yet (Dossey 1989, cited by

Olson et al 1992). Fedoruk (1985) therefore makes a helpful differentiation between two forms of administering the treatment: Therapeutic Touch *a*, where actual physical contact takes place between the practitioner and the recipient, and Therapeutic Touch *b*, where it does not.

Many researchers have studied 'touch' in nursing (e.g. McCorkle 1974, Weiss 1986) and one example of the many general definitions is, 'touch is the tactile stimulation of one person by another that is either planned or incidental' (Mulaik et al 1991). The technique of TT as introduced by Krieger, however, involves touching with the intent to help or heal by meditation (Krieger 1975, 1979) and is therefore not entirely synonymous with most general definitions of touch.

TT has been derived from the ancient practice of 'the laying on of hands' (Krieger 1975, Sherman 1985, Quinn 1989a) and Payne (1989) has clarified how it differs from this in five ways:

- the healer does not have to have religious beliefs

- the client does not have to have faith in TT

- it is knowledge based on research

- as a nursing intervention it is based on a specific assessment

- the afflicted individual has the potential to perform TT on himself or herself.

Green (1986) writes that there is a whole spectrum of healing therapies: touch and massage (e.g. Harrison 1986), TT, hand healing (done by people who believe that they have healing powers) and faith healing. The differences between the therapies are based on the belief systems of the healers and the clients. He gives as a minimal description of a healing ritual, '... a person holding and accepting another, both highly aware and attentive, awaiting some change.'

Finally, in searching for a definition of Therapeutic Touch, Quinn (1989a, 1992) reminds the reader that the fundamental focus is on healing and 'wholeness' rather than on disease or symptoms of disease. The word 'heal' derives from the Anglo-Saxon word 'haelan' meaning 'to become whole', or 'harmony of body–mind–spirit'. Quinn, finding the term to heal a definitional challenge, explains it by defining the opposite:

When we are alienated, isolated, estranged, fragmented, groundless, or rootless (from our bodies, our deepest self, culture, etc.) we are not whole; we are in a wrong relationship; we are diseased ... the elicitation of the haelan effect, the total organismic response towards wholeness, is the goal of Therapeutic Touch.

(Quinn 1992)

To summarise the main points so far, the treatment of TT has been described by most researchers and practitioners as a derivative of the laying on of hands, but a process that takes place outside a religious context. It is viewed as a natural human potential that can be accomplished by anyone who wishes to help or heal.

Similar terms such as faith-healing and hand-healing have been mentioned and, although not synonymous with the term, may have had some similarities in their origins. The next section therefore attempts to build on Chapter 1 and locate in the literature the historical development of TT from its ancient beginnings to the work of Krieger and successive researchers.

Ancient beginnings in religion

The earliest figure known for having healing powers by the laying on of hands was Imhotep, a court architect of King Zozer of the Third Egyptian Dynasty, about 2700 BC (Hodgkinson 1990, MacManaway & Turcan 1983). MacManaway & Turcan described how Imhotep was deified after his death and many temples were erected and dedicated to him where the sick were brought for healing. This healing cult spread via Persia to ancient Greece, where the god assumed the name of Asklepios. Asklepios was a Greek physician and spiritual healer who was also deified after his death. It is probable that the two cults are linked as Imhotep was thought to inhabit the body of a snake (MacManaway & Turcan 1983) and Asklepios (the patron saint of all physicians) has as his emblem a snake coiled round a rod, which is still the symbol of medicine (Hodgkinson 1990).

The term 'laying on of hands' for healing purposes is most commonly ascribed to the teachings and life of Jesus Christ (Zefron 1975). However, according to MacManaway & Turcan, what Jesus practised was not intrinsically new. They cite many authorities who argue that Mary and Joseph were Essenes (a sect who, according to the Roman historian Flavius Josephus, practised various forms of spiritual healing) and that Jesus received his early education in the *Therapeutae* temples in the years after fleeing from Herod. Chapter 1 shows how TT is viewed as a natural human potential. Zefron (1975) refers to passages in the Bible that show how Jesus commissioned his followers and regarded it as not out of the ordinary that they should be able to heal the sick (see, for example, Mark 9: 14–29, Luke 9: 37–41 and Matthew 17: 14–21).

Hodgkinson (1990) describes how in the Western world the concept of spiritual healing had 'virtually died' by the fourth century AD because there was a deeply held fear that occult practices such as witchcraft could be associated with healing, especially the type that seems to run counter to normal scientific rationale. For example:

> *'Until as late as 1951, I and others like me ran the theoretical risk of arrest under the Witchcraft Act which carried the death penalty, even if it had not been used for some time.'*
>
> (MacManaway & Turcan 1983)

In describing the history of TT, Turton (1988) cites one of the first Catholics involved in the recent 'charismatic renewal' of the Christian Church (MacNutt 1979), who maintains that there are three sources of healing power:

- the divine power of God
- demonic power
- a natural force of healing, based on love, which some people appear to have.

Turton explains that if this recognition of healing is a natural gift, it can absolve both the practitioner and the client from any guilty fear that they may be meddling in superstitious practices. Only one article in the nursing literature was found to discourage TT specifically on the grounds that it may be a superstitious practice, and for that reason it will be mentioned here. It was claimed by Miller (1987) that:

If one assumes the energy (the universal energy field) is the Holy Spirit
… the healer commits blasphemy by assuming a directive, manipulating
role with God himself. If on the other hand … the energy is some kind of
psychic power, then scripture forbids us to take part in it.

The above statement is valid in that it supports the teachings of
the New Testament, however Miller fails to explain clearly the differences between TT and faith healing, which is practised in the
Christian world. It is also unclear (due to the lack of literature)
whether the opinions expressed are representative of other Christian
and non-Christian nurses.

The historic assumption that all matter is surrounded by a universal life energy can be found in Brennan's (1988) review of the history
of healing through the human energy field. In the Old Testament there
are many accounts of light energy surrounding people, but over the
centuries the phenomena have lost their original meanings. For example, Michelangelo's statue of Moses depicts him with two horns on his
head, rather than the two beams of light, which the word 'karnaeem'
originally tried to convey. The confusion arose because this word can
mean either horn or light in Hebrew. Brennan cites White & Krippner
(1977), who listed 97 different cultures that refer to the human energy
field with 97 different names. In India, sacred writings refer to this life
energy as prana and in China since the third millennium BC it has
been named Qi (ch'i) (Brennan 1988, Hodgkinson 1990, Krieger 1975,
MacManaway & Turcan 1983, Talbot 1991, Turton 1988).

Finally, traditional Cree and other native American healing practices have also been linked with the concept of energy fields and
Krieger's (1979) technique of TT (Morse et al 1991). For particularly
serious cases of illness an Indian healer performs a ceremony where
dead eagle wings are used to intersect the eagle spirit, a healing
energy that surrounds a person.

The historic and religious concepts of TT such as the eagle ceremony may create healing energy in ways that from a fundamental
scientific view were not understood by the cultures that practised
them. The history of healing has a strong association with religion
and spiritual disciplines and can still be seen today in cultures that
have not abandoned their traditions. Could it be that the ancient

traditions of the world are simply different interpretations of the same phenomenon, whether it be a natural/learned human potential, superstitious practice or merely a placebo effect?

In the early 1960s the Canadian biochemist Bernard Grad conducted double-blind studies on the use of TT on mice and barley seeds, with the help of a renowned healer, Oskar Estabany. Krieger (1975), Clark & Clark (1984) and Turton (1988) all cite these studies and explain how they inspired Dolores Krieger in pioneering research and practice of TT in the nursing profession.

Early research

STUDIES ON MICE

Grad (1961) argued that if healing was the result of some energy force, rather than the power of suggestion, then it would have measurable effects on plants and animals. In his first study, Grad selected 300 standardised mice and marked their skin in a specific manner. One-third of the group was allowed to heal without any intervention and these were used as the control group. Estabany treated another 100 with the laying on of hands, and the remainder were held by medical students who claimed to have no healing abilities. According to Krieger (1975) after 2 weeks healing in Estabany's group had accelerated to a degree that could have happened by chance less than 1 in 1000 times. Turton (1988) also describes how Grad concluded that wound healing was definitely and significantly accelerated in those animals that had been held by the healer. Conversely Clark & Clark (1984), who provide long, detailed accounts and analyses of these experiments describe how only on the 15th and 16th days of study did the investigators find significantly smaller wound sizes for mice treated by the healer. On subsequent days their wound sizes were found to have no significant difference between mice treated by the healer and the control groups, and on completion of the study many mice not in the experimental group were found to have a similar degree of healing.

It must be pointed out here that Clark & Clark's article does not go beyond research completed after 1979. Furthermore, their discussion concerns research on the laying on of hands and on psychic healing, both of which are only peripherally related to TT. Neither of the studies mentioned in their article concerns research on human beings, and it is the effect on human beings that has been the sole focus of research on TT since the term was first coined by Krieger in 1974.

STUDIES ON SEEDS

In Grad's (1963) study on barley seedlings, the seeds were soaked in a saline solution to simulate a 'sick' condition (Krieger 1975). They were then divided into three groups, two controls and one experimental. The first control group was watered with tap water, the second with water from flasks held by disinterested persons and the third group was watered from flasks held by Estabany. The dependent variables were the number of plants per pot, the average height of plants per pot and plant yield per pot. Again according to Krieger (1975), the experimental seeds (those watered by Estabany) sprouted more quickly, grew taller and had more chlorophyll than the seeds in the control groups. Clark & Clark (1984), however, reported that data analysis by means of a t-test indicated that on only one day did the experimental group contain a significantly greater number of plants.

Grad's study on barley seeds did show some significant results, although they may have been biased because the healer prepared all pots and seeds before the experiment started. Grad's rationale was simply that he lacked personnel to carry out these tasks (Clark & Clark 1984). This threat to internal validity could have been reduced if Grad had employed another person to prepare the sample.

STUDIES ON ENZYMES

The biochemist Sister Justa Smith (1972) decided to test whether or not healing could positively affect the enzyme trypsin in solution. As with Grad, Oskar Estabany was used as the healer. Her assumption was that if enzyme failure is the ultimate physical cause of disease (as proposed by biomedical evidence), any therapeutic effect should be detectable at the same level. Her sample consisted of four solutions of trypsin. One was retained in its native state and used as a control, the second was treated by Estabany for 75 minutes by gripping the test-tube in which it was contained, the third was exposed to ultraviolet light and then treated by Estabany, and the fourth exposed to a magnetic field. Ultraviolet light possesses a wavelength that slightly denatures exposed trypsin, reducing its activity (Smith 1972).

It was concluded that the healer and magnetic field exerted similar positive effects on the enzyme, as the three solutions displayed an increase in enzyme activity. Although Smith reported standard deviations and means of the activity levels of the solutions, she did not calculate any statistical tests for the significance of the findings (Clark & Clark 1984). According to Smith, there was no difference between Estabany's effect on the native and the partially denatured enzyme. That is, both samples in response to Estabany's 'healing' showed an increase in enzyme activity. It is worth noting that the active site of an enzyme resides in a relatively small part of the molecule, and that a partially denatured enzyme can still function. It is possible that the increase of enzyme activity could have been attributed to the heat from Estabany's hands. Smith reported three replication studies of the experiment, but very few details with respect to any of the replications are discussed, and it is possible that the initial findings may have been due to chance.

It is unclear if Krieger (1975) was aware of the limitations of the Grad (1961, 1963) and Smith (1972) studies because they were not mentioned in her writings on them. Nevertheless, she described how, in the late 1960s and early 1970s, Oskar Estabany visited the United States for a few weeks each year to set up a temporary healing clinic with a well known observer of hand healing, Dora Kunz (Krieger 1975). Krieger observed the interactions with Estabany and the patients very closely, and explained how a significant number of them were cured physically, stating that:

Most of them had verified medical histories and had been referred by physicians who, when the patients returned for follow-up examination, confirmed their improvement.

(Krieger 1975)

It was these experiences that made Krieger decide to study TT in detail by conducting her own research within the nursing profession.

In exploring the related history of TT the literature has shown how healing practices were prominent in early societies, as they still are in many indigenous cultures today. Traditionally the concept has been interpreted from a religious perspective. However, the experiments of Grad (1965) and Smith (1972) demonstrate the growing interest that modern science has had in TT and that has led researchers to question the 'ultimate' cause of disease and health. For example, Smith (1972) pointed out that:

> *Without denying the initial premise that disease can be traced to a malfunctioning enzyme, the next question logically would be: what causes the enzyme to function improperly? Or what causes it ever again to function properly? When it comes to healing, we really do not know how even an aspirin works.*

To try and answer the question of how healing works, and to interpret the phenomenon of TT as a healing practice, nursing literature has developed a theoretical basis that covers aspects of nursing theory and modern science.

Is there a theoretical framework for Therapeutic Touch?

A theory has been defined as an 'intellectual invention designed to describe, explain, predict or prescribe' (Dickoff & James 1968). In other words, theories are not discovered but invented to understand phenomena. To date, practitioners, researchers and educators have used an energy field model as the theoretical framework for interpreting TT (Quinn 1989b). This theory postulates that the outcome of energy between healer and recipient can be deduced from the wider conceptual system proposed by Martha Rogers (1970, 1990) (see Chapter 3 for a more detailed discussion.) Rogers explained that people are open systems of energy, 'The human field extends beyond the discernible mass which we perceive as man. The human field and the environmental field ... are coextensive with the universe' (Rogers 1970). As noted in Chapter 1, the view that humans and the environment are inseparable is a fundamental component of ancient religions and Eastern philosophies.

When relating this assumption to TT, Quinn (1984) describes how when one person interacts with another there is an integration of energy fields and they become each other's immediate environment. If a change occurs in either person, it is considered to be an outcome of this field interaction. This change can be healing.

According to Miller (1979), this healing occurs through the interaction of the energy fields of man and environment whereby one field, 'actively works in the direction of change'. A particular human field 'healer' can have an environment, which is an integral part of an 'ill' human field.

TT can be viewed as a purposive patterning of the ill person's field in which the practitioner uses his or her hands as a meditating focus to promote healing (Meehan 1990a). The recipient's energies are then patterned so that they are, 'readily available to use in creating the necessary momentum toward health' (Boguslawski 1990), and this is achieved by the practitioner assuming a meditative state of awareness (Meehan 1990b), termed by Krieger (1979) as 'centring'.

Malinski (1991), in exploring Rogers' Science of Unitary Human Beings, hypothesises that the concept of spirituality is synonymous with the principle of integrality. In this view, spirituality as integrality is the belief in the notion of an underlying unity between man and the environment. Hover-Kramer (1990) explains further by saying that, 'we are in fact non-local in nature, connected with each other in mysterious ways as evidenced by the almost universal experiences of telepathy … and being influenced by others'. Centring during TT treatment heightens the experience of this integrality within the practitioner and the recipient (Malinski 1991).

ENERGY FIELDS

Rogers' (1970, 1990) conceptual system has described energy fields, yet it is important to have some concept of what a 'field' is. Boleman (1985) describes it as a space within which an action occurs. In the context of non-traditional forms of energy, the human field may partly consist of something called emotional energy (Wright 1991). Wright uses the example of anger, which can often be felt by another, even without the obvious presence of verbal or non-verbal language.

Perhaps, therefore, the practitioner's intention to help through centring can be felt by the person receiving Therapeutic Touch?

It is important to note here that there have been no reports that measure the interaction of energy fields to date (Quinn 1989b). However, the Rogerian premise of a human energy field integrated with an environmental energy field is well supported in the literature by modern scientific thought. Several mechanisms from physics – the science dealing with properties and interactions of matter and energy – apply to the understanding of Rogers' (1970) concepts, and these are summarised below:

Relativity

Perhaps the best known theory from modern physics is Einstein's Theory of Relativity. Einstein postulated that light has a constant velocity and this led to his famous equation relating mass to energy ($E = mc^2$), the basis of understanding atomic energy. This simple equation has some remarkable consequences when applied to the Rogerian concept, because it sums up the equivalence of energy and mass. In other words, mass and energy are interchangeable – two manifestations of the same reality. The basic substance of the universe according to Einstein is not matter but energy (Hawking 1988, Laffan 1993, Payne 1989).

Quantum theory

According to the laws of classical physics, if an object is warmed it should emit the same kind of blue–white light that it does when it is extremely hot. However, in reality it turns red. Max Planck discovered this principle in 1900 whilst investigating black-body radiation. This led him to announce his 'radiation law', according to which light was not emitted as a continuous flow as previously thought, but was made up of discrete units or 'quanta' of energy (Gribbon 1989).

This discovery was very significant in that it was the first evidence that the subatomic world behaves according to completely different post-Newtonian rules (Brazier 1992). The theory contradicted classical physics because it suggested that light was made of particles (quanta) instead of waves. Actually, physicists have since discovered that light can manifest as either particles or waves. An experiment by Thomas Young in 1803 proved that light was made up of waves by shining a light at a barrier with two slits in it. The light passed through the two slits and interference, which can only have occurred because the light was in the form of waves, created dark patches. Conversely, light can also be seen to be made of particles via Einstein's photoelectric experiment. Considering the same two-slit experiment as before, a single quantum of light can go through one slit and land in an area that would be dark if two slits were open. Physicists have wondered how the quantum knows whether the other slit is open or closed and some have even speculated that quanta may possess consciousness (Brazier 1992). There is also evidence that quanta only manifest as particles when they are being observed (Padmanabhan 1992). Talbot (1991) cites the physicist Nick Herbert, a supporter of this interpretation who states:

Humans can never experience the true texture of quantum reality because everything we touch or look at turns to matter.

The implication that all matter is an ambiguous 'soup' of quanta and appears as normal reality only when we are looking at it supports Rogers' theoretical system that humans are 'irreducible' energy fields integrated with each other and their environment.

Interconnectedness

Quantum theory showed how local reality may be true only at a certain level yet, according to Chopra (1990), the physicist John Bell developed this further by explaining that the reality of the whole universe is non-local. Bell's theorem shows by a famous mathematical equation that all objects and events are interconnected with each other and respond to one another's changes of state. This concept can be equated with Rogers' principle of integrality as discussed above.

To date, practitioners, teachers and researchers have used an energy model for explaining the phenomenon, and this has also been deduced from the Rogerian conceptual system of the Science of

Unitary Human Beings. The energy model has support from advances in modern physics, which show that on the subatomic level the classical laws of physics do not apply and that the universe may well consist of interconnected energy of which life is a part.

Research on Therapeutic Touch

When applying the conceptual system of Rogers' Science of Unitary Human Beings (1990) to research studies, the question being asked is: 'How does the outcome of a study have an effect?' No published studies directly measuring energy exchange have been found in the literature, therefore to apply the theory to current research, the logical consequences of the theory have to be scrutinised.

Quinn (1989b) suggests six general assumptions that need to be verified in TT research:

1. there is a human energy field, which is primary and not secondary to biochemical physiologic processes

2. in illness there is an imbalance in the energy field (the term 'imbalance' should be operationalised)

3. energy moves between human fields

4. energy can be 'sent' from one person to another

5. 'recipient' of this energy alters the field of the recipient

6. if energy can be transferred, it impacts on the health of the recipient.

Therefore, in reviewing TT research, this critique will include an enquiry into the logical consequences and conceptual limitations of studies that are applicable to one or more of the assumptions laid down by Quinn (1989a), in addition to looking at methodological issues such as research design.

HAEMOGLOBIN

The work of Dr Dolores Krieger in 1974 was the first scientific attempt to study the effects of TT using trained registered nurses.

Krieger (1975, 1979) used an Eastern philosophical view of health to conceptualise this pioneering research, whereby a healthy person has an overabundance of energy, or prana (see Chapter 1), and a deficit of this causes illness. Krieger felt that:

Prana can be activated by will and can be transferred to another person if one has the intent to do so. The literature also states that prana is intrinsic in what we would call one oxygen molecule.

(Krieger 1975)

It was postulated that a trained TT practitioner could activate and facilitate the flow of this healing energy. Krieger's reasoning for choosing haemoglobin was that she claimed it was one of the most sensitive indicators of oxygen uptake (Krieger 1975). Krieger also reasoned that haemoglobin's similarity to chlorophyll was another reason for its selection. She reported that Grad's studies on barley seeds, 'showed an increase in the chlorophyll content of the sample that had been irrigated by Estabany ... and that chlorophyll and haemoglobin have a similar "stereochemical structure".' She further reasoned that the selection of haemoglobin would be appropriate for a dependent variable, as haemoglobin is closely associated with the functioning of several enzymes. This deduction was based on Smith's (1972) findings on enzyme activity discussed earlier. Krieger took a convenience sample of 32 nurses out of 75 who asked to participate. The 32 selected nurses were those who Krieger believed best showed the qualities of a 'humanistic nurse', and they were taught methods of TT either by Krieger or by her colleague Dora Kunz. Each trained nurse was asked to choose one patient to receive TT and a second to receive routine care. The sample therefore comprised of 64 hospitalised patients, half of whom were treated with TT (the experimental group), and half given routine care.

The results, which were supported by Fisher's *t*-test for the comparison of correlated means, showed a statistically significant increase in post-test haemoglobin values in those patients in the experimental group. The hypothesis that the haemoglobin levels of those patients would change significantly from their pre-test values was therefore supported.

Methodological problems

The reasoning behind using haemoglobin as the dependent variable warrants criticism, as haemoglobin is not a measure of oxygen uptake, but a measure of oxygen capacity. It has been suggested that an appropriate measure of oxygen uptake would have been the oxygen saturation of blood (Clark & Clark 1984). Krieger's assumptions, based on Grad's (1961, 1963) and Smith's (1972) studies, are also questionable because Grad (1963) did not use chlorophyll as a dependent measure in his study and Smith did not report testing for statistical difference between pre- and post-experiment measures of enzyme activity.

Absence of operational definitions and random group assignment further weaken Krieger's (1975) study, although she did report using a *t*-test to establish the comparability of haemoglobin levels between groups. The *t*-test is a powerful parametric test and is the classic technique for analysing the differences between the means of two groups, thus one of the assumptions it has to meet is that there are equal variances between these groups (Brink & Wood 1989). As Krieger (1975) did not report the manner in which the hospital patients were chosen, the significant results have to be treated with caution, because homogeneity in terms of age, sex and type of illness cannot be assumed.

THE RELAXATION RESPONSE

Further collaborative work by Krieger and colleagues (Kreiger et al 1979) reported the first 'evidence' of a deep relaxation state being present in clients receiving TT. This was verified by objective electronic measurements of dependent physiological variables of three patients and a healer (Krieger) during TT. Electroencephalographic and galvanic skin responses were measured for all participants; electromyographic and electro-oculographic responses for the healer were noted; and the patients' electrocardiogram (ECG) and hand temperature were recorded.

The EEG results of the healer demonstrated a predominant amount of fast synchronous beta activity during the procedures, which was interpreted as indicating a state of deep concentration:

On analysing the data, it can be considered that the rapid synchronous beta activity in Krieger's EEG represents the physiological style of TT that ... can be considered to be in actuality a healing meditation.

(Krieger et al 1979)

The electro-ocular records of the healer collected during her administration of TT showed that her eyes had 'no movement', which was interpreted by Krieger et al (1979) as an indicator of her steady concentration during the procedure.

Collected data from the patients indicated that there was a high amount of large amplitude alpha activity while their eyes were open. According to the authors this indicated a deep state of relaxation because, 'aside from a study done on Zen Buddhist masters, the alpha state is usually accomplished in the closed eyes state by most people' (Krieger et al 1979).

No other significant results were recorded and it is unclear as to why the healer and patients did not have the same physiological variables measured for comparability. In addition, data and statistical tests were not reported in the text. This challenges the credibility of the study, and the conclusions therefore have to be viewed with caution.

The work of Krieger et al (1979) served as a bridge between TT and the relaxation response for at least ten other researchers who studied the effect of TT on either anxiety or stress (Fedoruk 1984, Gagne & Toye 1994, Garrard 1995, Heidt 1981, Olson & Sneed 1995, Olson et al 1992, Olsen et al 1997, Parkes 1985, Quinn 1984, Quinn 1989b, Randolph 1984).

CONTROLLING THE PLACEBO PHENOMENON

Any procedure that produces an effect in a patient because of its therapeutic intent and not its specific nature is called a placebo (Liberman 1962). For example 'fake' drugs can cause the adrenal glands to secrete and the stomach's blood flow to increase (Wolf 1950), therefore it appears possible that placebos can produce objective physical changes. As the nature of TT is hypothesised as an energy exchange that lies within the wider concepts of Rogerian science, it would appear pertinent that when subjective symptoms of subjects are being studied the inclusion of a placebo control group (under double-blind conditions) is essential to eliminate the possibility of a placebo effect.

The research design of Heidt's (1981) study, which claimed that hospitalised patients who received TT had significantly lower levels of state anxiety (a transitory emotional state characterised by a subjective, consciously perceived feeling of tension, apprehension and heightened autonomic nervous system activity (Quinn 1984, 1989b)), highlights the above proposal. Heidt logically reasoned that if TT could influence levels of physiological relaxation as in Krieger et al's (1979) study, it could also influence the level of anxiety experienced by a subject. A total of 90 hospitalised cardiovascular patients, who had volunteered for the study, were randomised into three groups. The experimental group received TT by a practitioner for 5 minutes. Another group, the control group, received casual touch for 5 minutes (this consisted of a nurse taking various pulses from each subject). The third group received no intervention by touch, but instead had a nurse who sat and talked to the patient for 5 minutes. This was designed as a control for the effect of the presence of another helping person.

Pre- and post-treatment anxiety levels were assessed using the Self-evaluation Questionnaire (Spielberger et al 1970), which, on comparison of pre-test and post-test means, demonstrated a statistically significant decrease in state anxiety in the experimental group. This group also had a statistically significant greater reduction in state anxiety scores than the other two groups when analyses of covariance were performed on the data. This test was a more suitable method than Krieger's (1975) use of multiple tests because it meant that post-test means could be adjusted to account for pre-test differences of state anxiety.

It is questionable as to whether the research design of Heidt's (1981) study allowed for TT to be interpreted as a major factor in the reduction of anxiety because there was no control for the placebo effect. Subjects had received different types of behavioural stimulation and had known when TT was being administered to them. The hypothesised energy transfer in this case therefore could not be tested.

MIMIC THERAPEUTIC TOUCH

The first research to expose two groups to what appeared to be the same treatment was Randolph's (1984) study on the physiological responses of female college students to stressful stimuli whilst receiving TT. Randolph (1984) built on the previous work of Krieger et al (1979), which claimed that TT produced a relaxation response. Randolph (1984) took this reasoning further by hypothesising that the physiological stress response of persons treated with imitated TT would exceed the physiological stress response of persons treated with genuine TT.

A film entitled *Subincision* served as a stressful stimulus. This was a silent footage film showing a sequence of operations performed on tribal adolescent boys. An experimental group of 30 subjects received TT and a control group of 30 subjects received imitated treatment. Whilst they watched the film they were simultaneously monitored for signs of anxiety – muscle tension, galvanic skin resistance and temperature were measured as indicators of state anxiety.

No significant differences in the post-treatment dependent variables were reported and both groups responded to the film with a recognisably similar amount of stress. This might be viewed as a lack of support for the contextual theory that energy exchange is the means by which TT has an effect, as both groups received the same behavioural stimulus. The study was also the first published investigation that was double blind in design – neither the subject nor the data collector were informed of the subject's group assignment until after the session. Although TT was performed by nurses who had been trained to administer the treatment, the question arose as to how the level of ability that had been achieved by the TT practitioners could be validated. Randolph (1984) suggested that TT research would benefit from the development of a tool to address this problem.

It has been suggested that the main factor that produced the non-significant results was the level of health of the subjects (Randolph 1984). Randolph used healthy college students, whilst previous research (Heidt 1981, Krieger 1975) employed less healthy subjects. As the stress response is a normal physiological process, which protects the person from external threats, then perhaps TT would be unable to suppress such a response.

This issue arises again in later research by Rosalie Fedoruk (1984, 1985), who studied the effect of TT and a mimic treatment on the response to stress in neonates in intermediate and intensive care. Fedoruk's unpublished doctoral dissertation sought to answer the question of whether Therapeutic Touch *b* (non-contact) would reduce the stress of the nursing procedure of measuring 'vital signs' in premature infants. The outcome measures of infant state and transcutaneous oxygen blood gas pressure ($TcPO_2$) were used to measure stress.

Quinn (1988) cited no rationale for Fedoruk's choice of transcutaneous oxygen blood gas pressure as a dependent variable and therefore it is presumed from the text that higher levels of $TcPO_2$ correspond with greater levels of relaxation and oxygen uptake. Fedoruk's reasoning may also have been influenced by Krieger's (1975) studies on haemoglobin values, which postulated that the energy transferred during TT is bound to the oxygen molecule. Infant state was measured using the Assessment of Premature Infant Behaviour (APIB) scale.

A convenience sample of 17 premature neonates was studied and each infant received each of the interventions twice. Repeated measures analysis of covariance were used to test the hypotheses. These analyses showed that infants treated with TT demonstrated a greater change from a higher, more aroused, state to a lower, more relaxed, state during the observation time than infants receiving mock TT or no TT.

No statistical differences were found between $TcPO_2$ levels between groups, indicating that TT had no effect on the physiological indicators of stress.

Fedoruk warned that the results could not be interpreted with any degree of certainty. The cautions conveyed in Fedoruk's study were highlighted by Quinn (1988), and included:

■ the sample size of 17 was too small

■ the treatment times were not equal; Therapeutic Touch lasted for 5 minutes whereas the control treatments lasted for 1 minute.

As in Randolph's (1984) study, the issue of whether TT should suppress the appropriate response to external stressors arises again:

> *When one examines the major assumptions of the study … one finds that relaxation is seen as the equivalent of suppressing reactivity to real stressors in the external environment.*
>
> (Quinn 1988)

It is probably, therefore, a healthy and normal response for an infant to react to stimuli in the environment as Randoph's research demonstrated, and it is unlikely that TT would suppress such a response.

MIMIC THERAPEUTIC TOUCH AND SUBJECTIVE STATE ANXIETY

Support for the hypothesis of energy transfer depends on how well controlled studies are. It has already been shown that there is a need to control for the placebo phenomenon. Indeed it has sometimes been difficult to reflect the results back to the theory (e.g. Krieger 1979, Heidt 1981), because the studies have not been derived directly from the Rogerian conceptual system. This theory testing was addressed directly by Quinn (1984) and Parkes (1985) and replicated by Quinn (1989b).

The studies utilised subjective state anxiety as a measure of the efficacy of TT because the effect of TT on state anxiety had already been researched (Heidt 1981). Mimic TT (originally called non-contact TT) was operationally defined for the first time by Quinn (1982) as:

> *…an intervention which mimics the movements of the nurse during TT, but during which there is no attempt to centre, no intention to assist the subject, no attuning to the condition of the subject, and no direction of energy.*

TT in these three studies was practised without using physical contact, as it was reasoned that physical contact would not be needed if TT involved a type of energy exchange. This treatment was defined as non-contact Therapeutic Touch.

State anxiety was defined as a transitory emotional state or condition of the human organism that is characterised by a subjective, consciously perceived feeling of tension, apprehension and heightened autonomic nervous system activity (Quinn 1984, 1989b). This was measured by a Self-Evaluation Questionnaire, STAI (State Trait Anxiety Inventory) form, developed by Spielberger, Gorsuch and Lushene (Spielberger 1970).

In the first study, Quinn (1982, 1984) randomly assigned a convenience sample of 60 hospitalised adults with cardiovascular disease to either a group receiving TT or a group receiving the mimic treatment. Three nurses who had no knowledge of TT carried out these mimic interventions. All subjects completed a STAI questionnaire before and after the study. Both treatments lasted for approximately 5 minutes.

The findings of Quinn's (1982) study supported the hypothesis that there would be a greater decrease in post-test state anxiety scores in subjects treated with non-contact TT than mimic TT. This was supported at the 0.0005 level of significance, lending confidence to the theorem that TT involved an energy exchange.

However in a doctoral dissertation by Parkes (1985, cited by Quinn 1988) the effect of TT on the state anxiety of gerontological hospitalised patients was studied. It was found that there were no significant differences in reduction of anxiety in the group that received TT from the control groups. This study used a similar research design to Quinn's (1982), except there was an additional control group where the treatment nurse held her hands over the shoulder area of the subjects. Three groups of 20 hospitalised elderly patients between the ages of 65 and 93 years had completed the STAI questionnaire before and after the study, and the comparison of post-test means using analysis of covariance had revealed no differences that were statistically significant.

Finally, Quinn's replication of her 1982 study (Quinn 1989b), like Parkes' (1985) study, also failed to support the energy exchange hypothesis. This replication differed from her first study, which had supported the conceptual theory, by one major factor: the mimic TT treatment was administered without eye contact. Quinn's derived theorem from the Rogerian conceptual system was that eye contact would not be needed for TT to be effective. In fact the significant results of her last study could have been related to some form of subtle communication such as facial cues from the practitioner.

Quinn's replication study (Quinn 1989b) used a sample of 38 women and 115 men who were hospitalised awaiting open-heart surgery on the following day. As in the original study (Quinn 1982), the STAI questionnaire was used to measure state anxiety. The dependent variables of blood pressure and heart rate were also measured on each subject and pre- and post-test measures were tested using separate analyses of covariance. No significant differences were recorded in any of the variables for those subjects who were treated by TT or those who received the mimic treatment.

The negative findings of Quinn's (1989b) and Parkes's (1985) studies might thus be viewed as lack of support for the Rogerian conceptual theory by which TT may have an effect. If eye contact is needed, it may be possible that some form of placebo action is in operation, whereby the recipient of TT can 'sense' the practitioner's intent to help them.

However, methodological designs combined with contextual factors also need to be taken into account for the interpretation of results. Unlike Quinn's original (1982) study, the nurse in the replication study (Quinn 1989b) provided both TT and mimic TT. Meditation and 'intentionality' are intrinsic to the TT process. It may therefore be possible that meditation and the purpose of intent cannot be turned on or off by conscious choice or will by the experienced practitioner. Quinn (1989b) supported this notion by explaining that it is possible to be in two states of consciousness at the same time, for example when driving a car. This may have explained the closeness of results in both groups.

Although the results in Quinn's (1989b) study were not significant, all post-test measures did change in the predicted direction, with the largest changes occurring in the TT group. Quinn suggested that premature ending of the treatment might have resulted in failure of the dependent variable changes to reach significance because the treatment had only lasted for 5 minutes.

IS EYE CONTACT NEEDED FOR THERAPEUTIC TOUCH?

The negative findings of Quinn's (1989b) replicate study can be inter-preted as suggesting that eye and facial contact are necessary for TT to have an effect and that therefore a mechanism other than energy exchange is responsible, such as the placebo phenomenon.

However, if further investigations demonstrate that eye and facial contact are important, this would still not rule out that energy exchange is responsible for TT. Brennan (1988) explained that the eyes can be used for a powerful focus of energy and therefore absence of such contact may hinder the healing process.

Although no other research has investigated facial contact during TT, the hypothesis that the eyes may help facilitate this energy exchange might be supported by one of the very few qualitative studies to investigate TT. An as yet unpublished study by France (1991) used a multiple perspective approach to discover the essence of a child's perception of TT. Phenomenology was the guiding philos-ophy for the selected methods and design, which included serial videotaped interview sessions, children's drawings, parental journals and the researcher's journal.

Eleven children aged three to nine years were given TT. Phenomenological reduction and analysis of the data discovered an emerging theme of unity between the subjects, which was described by the researcher as 'that look'. The researcher captured this unity in the metaphor, 'the eyes tell all'. It appears that the eyes of the practitioner may have left an impression on the chil-dren while they received TT. It could have conveyed the desire or intent to help and may have supported the idea that eyes are a factor in concentrating energy or aiding intentionality. This could be further supported by electro-ocular records of a healer in Krieger's second published study (Krieger et al 1979), which showed no eye movement, indicative of a high level of concentration in the healer.

DISTANCE HEALING AS ENERGY EXCHANGE

The work of Beutler et al (1988) deserves a mention as one of the few experimental trials on TT to be carried out by non-nurses. The study sought to discover whether the laying on of hands and distance healing by a renowned healer could reduce hypertension.

Distance healing, whereby the healer 'transmits' healing to an individual who may be many miles away, is practised by some TT practitioners in North America and the UK (MacManaway & Turcan 1983). Within the context of Rogerian science, where humans and environment are considered as integrated energy fields interconnected with each other, it may be postulated that a healer and recipient could exchange energy whilst not being in immediate proximity to each other.

Beutler et al (1988) randomised patients into three treatment groups: healing by the laying on of hands ($n=40$), healing at a distance ($n=40$), and no healing (controls, $n=38$). Healing at a distance and no healing were investigated double blind.

It was reported that diastolic blood pressure fell in all three groups from week to week during the period of the trial, and that this was probably caused by a placebo effect of the trial itself. The researchers concluded that no treatment was consistently better than another, and therefore the data could not be taken as evidence of a paranormal effect on blood pressure.

The phenomenon of distance healing and energy exchange (but see also Chapter 1) would therefore appear not to be supported. However, the data study by Beutler et al (1988) did record that each week diastolic pressure was consistently lower in patients treated by healing at a distance than in those in the control group. Although paired comparisons yielded no significant differences, both groups were investigated under double blind conditions and therefore the reduction in the predicted direction may possibly have indicated a paranormal influence such as energy exchange.

THE EFFECT OF THERAPEUTIC TOUCH ON PAIN

To date, several studies have investigated the effects of TT on the experience of pain, and these have presented conflicting results.

Meehan (1990a) and Barrington (1994) examined whether TT was effective in decreasing pain in postoperative patients and Keller & Bzdek (1986) investigated its effects on tension headache. Both researchers built on previous work, which had indicated that TT had decreased anxiety (Heidt 1981, Quinn 1984), and reasoned that because anxiety influences the pain experience (Hayward 1975), TT should decrease pain. Meehan (1990a) hypothesised that subjects treated by TT would have a greater decrease in post-test acute pain than subjects treated by mimic TT. She also investigated whether the effects of TT would decrease pain more than standard treatment. Neither hypothesis was supported and it was found that the standard treatment of giving medication was significantly more effective than the administration of TT.

Keller & Bzdek (1986) hypothesised that subjects who received TT would experience greater headache relief than subjects who received mimic TT, and that their pain reduction would still be greater 4 hours after the treatment. This hypothesis was supported by statistically significant results of post-test scores, which dropped an average of 70% in the TT group and 37% in the control group.

Both research designs were rigorous, using operational definitions of treatments and time length (5 minutes), pain scale questionnaires and suitable data analysis tests. However, Meehan (1990a) used a large sample size of 108 subjects, whereas Keller & Bzdek's (1986) sample size was 60, which may have accounted for the statistical differences. Meehan also explained that a very conservative statistical test for significance was used (multiple regression analysis with post-hoc comparison of means) and that a less rigorous measure would in fact have supported her hypothesis. Like Quinn's (1989b) study on anxiety, the post-test measures of pain in this study did change in the predicted direction.

In 1998 Gordon et al did a single-blind, randomized control trial to determine if TT was effective in the treatment of osteoarthritis of the knee. It was concluded that, despite small numbers (25), significant differences were found in improvement in function and pain for patients receiving TT.

The results of these pain studies therefore appear to support the hypothesis that perhaps TT can relieve pain. The research designs, which were double blind and included a mimic treatment, also support the Rogerian conceptual theory of energy exchange by the logical consequences of results.

EFFECTS OF THERAPEUTIC TOUCH ON WOUND HEALING

The acceleration of wound healing with the use of TT has been researched by Wirth and colleagues (Wirth 1990, Wirth et al 1993, 1996). In the original randomised, double-blind study, 46 volunteers were divided into two groups – one control group and one group who received TT. All received a punch biopsy to their arms. The wounds were measured at regular intervals and the end results indicated a remarkable significant increase in the rate of healing in the TT group. A replication study (Wirth et al 1993) showed unequivocally that the TT subjects experienced a significant acceleration in the rate of wound healing compared to the control group subjects on day 5 and day 10 of the study. However, the 1996 study, where a randomised, double-blind methodological protocol was used to replicate the research above, found the results going in the opposite direction from that hypothesised (Wirth et al 1996). This is an important study as it is the first of its kind to indicate an inhibitory effect taking place when subjects were unaware of the physical and psychological state of the healer.

LENGTH OF TREATMENT FOR THERAPEUTIC TOUCH

Predetermining the TT treatment time for 5 minutes works very well in terms of operationally defining the intervention for research purposes (Quinn 1989a). It has worked well in producing significant outcomes for Heidt (1981), Quinn (1984) and Keller & Bzdek (1986).

However, Meehan (1990a) reported that in her pain study, 5 minutes may not have been long enough for an analgesic effect. As the decrease in pain in the TT group was very close to being significant, it may be reasonable to assume that a longer treatment time may have produced a greater effect against pain.

The poor results of the replicate study of anxiety (Quinn 1989b) were also attributed partly to this problem:

There were many sessions when the treatment nurse sensed that the treatment was just beginning to have an effect and that if a few more minutes were permitted the subject would indeed have been more relaxed.

(Quinn 1989b)

While this cannot be regarded as the main reason for the failure of Quinn's results, it is to be expected that some individuals would respond to TT more quickly than others, who would therefore require longer treatment.

A preliminary study, which sought to answer questions about the effectiveness of TT in reducing post-traumatic stress for 23 individuals (Olson et al 1992), addressed this methodological issue. This research was implemented in the 2 months that followed Hurricane Hugo in the United States with a convenience sample of volunteers who had experienced personal stress. Stress was confirmed by a short questionnaire that addressed the effects of the hurricane on their lives.

A repeated session design was used with data collected before, during and after each session, with heart rate, blood pressure and skin temperature used as the physiological dependent measures. The psychological dependent variables were state and trait anxiety, which were measured by two visual analogue scale questionnaires. State anxiety was defined in the study as how much stress the subject felt at that time, and trait anxiety as how much general stress the subject felt most days of his or her life.

The first two sessions were identical in that TT was administered by an experienced practitioner, who terminated the treatment at varying times according to 'subjective cues' from the client. The third session was a control session where the subject and healer sat quietly for 20 minutes in close proximity to each other.

The findings demonstrated that mean state anxiety scores decreased significantly after the TT sessions and also when compared to the control group. However, there were no significant differences in pre- and post-test trait anxiety scores. Physiological outcomes reflected relaxation trends but were not significantly different between treatment and control groups. Repeated measures of covariance were used to test these differences.

The decrease in state anxiety and length of treatment was significantly correlated with session length, which ranged from 6.8 minutes to 20 minutes, and suggests that perhaps future research on TT should allow more time for the healer to administer treatment.

Some of the limitations of this study by Olson et al (1992) were that the sample size was relatively small compared with previous research. Lack of randomisation and the small number of subjects that returned for the control sessions further weakened the results.

It is interesting from a contextual viewpoint that the control session in this study was similar to Heidt's (1981), whereby the healer sat by the patient for a specific amount of time. It is unclear why Olson et al (1992) abandoned the mimic treatment as a suitable control. Their reasoning was that their method:

> ...allowed the subject and toucher to be in the same environmental field without activity and avoided the mimic treatment criticised as confounding the results of other studies, for example Quinn (1989b).

Quinn (1989b) in her replicate anxiety study suggested, however, that persons not experienced in TT are the best candidates for mimic TT practitioners, because they would not drift into a consciousness of 'sending energy'.

A placebo effect may have accounted for the significant results of the investigation by Olson et al (1992), because the subjects received two different forms of behavioural stimulation from the healer. The theory of energy exchange can therefore not be supported from this study.

THE AGE FACTOR AND THE EFFECTIVENESS OF THERAPEUTIC TOUCH

There is evidence from at least two studies in the literature to suggest that older people are less responsive to TT (Parkes 1985, Quinn 1984). Quinn's (1982, 1994) study on anxiety found a low correlation between age and response to TT, such that it appeared that the older the subject the less post-test anxiety decreased. The results of Parkes's (1985) investigation were also consistent with these results. However, Quinn (1988) urged caution in interpreting the results by questioning the appropriateness of the STAI questionnaire for older people. This becomes more evident when one examines Parkes's (1985) study on hospitalised elderly patients, which reported that many of the subjects were concerned with trying to remember the answers from the pre-test.

A single-subject design investigating the effects of TT on the quality of sleep of elderly nursing home residents found that five out of six of the subjects had a better quality of sleep during nights when TT had been administered to them at bedtime (Braun et al 1986). Quality of sleep was measured using the Sleep Quality Questionnaire. The findings appeared to confirm that TT was effective in enhancing the sleep quality of elderly people. It was suggested by the authors that this technique be added to nursing measures used to help the elderly.

Rather than compare the effect of TT on groups of subjects, this study used a single-subject design, which meant that each individual acted as their own control. One of the advantages of single-subject designs is that they can be carried out using a small sample.

The authors did not describe any limitations to their study. However when examining the problem from an energy exchange viewpoint, the possibility of a placebo response cannot be eliminated, as residents were aware which evenings TT had been administered to them. Perhaps future single-subject designs could be double blind, for example in this study residents could have had TT administered to them once they were asleep and could also have been doubly unaware of which nights these were.

THE NEED FOR QUALITATIVE RESEARCH

With, for example, the exception of the study by France (1991), most of the research reviewed in this chapter has used a quantitative approach to investigating the TT phenomenon. Braun's sleep study, however, was pioneering, in that it was the first published research to approach the subject from a more qualitative direction. TT has been described as a deeply personal experience for both the practitioner and the patient (Heidt 1991). The study by Braun et al highlights the need for more single-subject designs and qualitative measures in quantitative designs, in order that the personal experience of TT can be investigated. New questions may emerge from such studies, which may stimulate and develop the theory of TT within the Rogerian worldview.

To date, only one other published TT research study has included qualitative measures within its design. The investigation of the effects of TT on post-traumatic stress by Olson et al (1992) included a collection of qualitative data that addressed the question of whether the person administering TT and the person receiving it agreed about the body locations where sensations related to TT were perceived.

A figure form with front and back line drawings of the human body was used after each treatment, on which both subject and healer, independently, marked any places on the figure that corresponded to sensations on the subject's body perceived during the treatment. Krieger (1979) had suggested that the figure form would be a useful tool for students in TT, but there are no records of reliability for this method in the research literature.

The results recorded a mean of only 13% agreement between subject and healer of where the sensations were felt on the subject's body. However, comments about the nature of their sensations ranged from 'nothing felt' to 'tingling' in both subjects and healer. The researchers reported many similarities when such comments between healer and subject were juxtaposed. This may be useful for later research in developing alternative tools to determine the interaction experience between healer and subject during TT.

The only wholly qualitative published study on TT was by Heidt in 1990 (although Lionberger had completed an unpublished doctoral dissertation in 1985). Using an inductive approach she analysed nurses' and patients' experiences of TT. A comparative method of data analysis from interviews and observations of seven nurse TT practitioners and seven subjects found that in many instances the experiences of the patients during the treatment paralleled those of the nurses.

When nurses had the inner experience of themselves as patterns of energy, which by nature are 'wholes' rather than 'parts', the patients reflected that shift in experience as well. Similarly, as the nurses stilled themselves and projected that sense of calm to the patient, the patient's energy stilled and they focused on the inner healing process. This 'transfer of energy' took place on a physical as well as psychological level (Heidt 1990).

The growing number of case studies on TT in the literature also provides a valuable qualitative type of indication of the experiences of patients and nurses. An analysis of these studies is beyond the scope of this literature review, although a complete list (to date) is available in the bibliography.

One such case study, which put forward a comparative review of sessions where two patients were treated by a TT practitioner (Heidt 1991), concluded that the patient who suffered from state anxiety was more amenable to treatment than the patient who suffered from trait anxiety. This reflected the results of the study by Olson et al (1992) of post-traumatic stress, which found similar results for the effects of TT on trait and state anxiety. This demonstrates the importance specific case studies can have in furthering the knowledge base of the phenomenon.

In 1999, Winstead-Fry and Kijek performed an integrative research review and meta-analysis of Therapeutic Touch research. This review demonstrated that:

- there are many approaches to Therapeutic Touch research

- samples are described incompletely

- the Therapeutic Touch practices vary in the studies. Most of the studies supported hypotheses regarding the efficacy of therapeutic touch, although a number had mixed or negative results.

Conclusion

In examining TT literature and research this review has shown how interest in the treatment has grown since its introduction into nursing in 1974. In searching for definitions of the phenomenon, it has been suggested that TT can be regarded as a natural potential, which any person could perform. TT is a contemporary interpretation of ancient healing practices, yet remains outside a religious context. The early experiments by Grad (1963) and Smith (1972) influenced Krieger to study the concept further and introduce it to the nursing profession. Nursing theory has attempted to explain the method, using an energy exchange model within the wider framework of the Rogerian world-view. Finally, a critique of nursing literature has been presented which highlights a number of issues. The theoretical context behind the studies has remained consistent yet the testing of the energy exchange theory remains inconclusive. An attempt has been made to apply the theory logically to research by examining the research designs and the consequences of their results. If practitioners and researchers continue to use Roger's Science of Unitary Human Beings (1970) to describe and explain TT, it is important that more research tests this theory directly, as Quinn (1984, 1989a, b) and Parkes (1985) did. The main issue that has arisen from this theory testing is the appropriateness of certain controls for the placebo response, as it appears important that subjects receive the same behavioural stimulus. It may also be pertinent to question whether what has been described as the placebo response is itself a re-patterning of a subject's energy field, which helps them regain health. This highlights the need for inter-disciplinary research to validate the existence of such an energy field.

Out of the 12 experimental studies analysed in this critique, only seven presented any type of result showing benefits from TT. The need for replication and further developments and improvement in research designs will substantiate what can so far be regarded as only preliminary 'proof' that TT can improve a person's health. Qualitative research may address this problem by exploring the phenomenon on a more personal level, yet to date this is lacking.

It is hoped that this literature review has presented the strengths and shortcomings of what is still a relatively unresearched subject. It needs to be pointed out, however, that tentative empirical support for TT should be no reason to discourage the practice. Many people have voiced an increased wellbeing from the treatment, evidenced from the number of case studies on the phenomenon, and there are no reports showing it to be harmful (Haviland 1986).

In 1975, Krieger implied TT was the hallmark of nursing (Krieger 1975) because it is an intrinsic attribute of the profession that almost every nursing skill is performed with the act of touch. It may be argued further that TT is the hallmark of nursing and other health care practitioners because the essence of the phenomenon is the intent of the one helping with healing to focus completely on the wellbeing of a patient. This process of unconditional love or positive regard may be the most quintessential act of caring a practitioner can perform.

REFERENCES

Barrington R 1994 A naturalistic inquiry of post-operative pain after therapeutic touch. In Gaut D A, Boykin A (eds) Caring as healing: renewal through hope. National League for Nursing, New York, pp 199–213

Beutler J J, Attevelt J T, Schouton S A, Faber J A, Mees E J, Geijskes G G 1988 Paranormal healing and hypertension. British Medical Journal 296:1491–1494

Boguslawski M 1990 Unitary human field practice modalities. In: Barret E A M (ed) Visions of Rogers' science based nursing. National League for Nursing, New York

Boleman J 1985 An introduction to physics. Prentice Hall, Englewood Cliffs

Braun C, Layton C J, Braun J 1986 Therapeutic Touch improves residents' sleep. American Health Care Association Journal 12(1):48–49

Brazier C 1992 An investigation into the paranormal. New Internationalist 237:4–7

Brennan B A 1988 Hands of light: a guide to healing through the human energy field. Bantam, London

Brink P J, Wood M J 1989 Basic steps in planning nursing research: from question to proposal. Jones and Bartlett, Boston

Carruthers A M 1992 A force to promote bonding and well being. Professional Nurse 7(5):297–300

Chopra D 1990 Quantum healing. Bantam, London

Clark P E, Clark M J 1984 Therapeutic Touch: is there a scientific basis for the practice? Nursing Research 33(1):37–41

Dickoff J, James P 1968 A theory of theories: a position paper. Nursing Research 17:197–203

Dossey L 1989 Recovering the soul: a scientific and spiritual search. Bantam, New York

Fedoruk R B 1984 Transfer of the relaxation response. Doctoral Dissertation, University of Maryland. Cited in Quinn J F 1988 Building a body of knowledge. Journal of Holistic Nursing 6(1):37–45

Fedoruk R B 1985 Transfer of the relaxation response: Therapeutic Touch as a method for reduction of stress in premature neonates. Dissertation Abstracts International 46:978

France M N E 1991 A phenomenological inquiry on the child's lived experience of perceiving the human energy field using Therapeutic Touch. Dissertation Abstracts International 52(12):6315–6316

Gagne D, Toye R 1994 The effects of therapeutic touch and relaxation therapy in reducing anxiety. Archives of Psychiatric Nursing 8(3):184–189

Garrard CT 1995 The effects of therapeutic touch on stress reduction and immune function in persons with AIDS. Dissertation Abstracts International 56(3692B). University microfilms no. 9537117

Gordon A, Merenstein J, D'Amico F, Hudgens D 1998 The effects of Therapeutic Touch on patients with osteoarthritis of the knee. The Journal of Family Practice 47(4):271–277

Grad B 1961 An unorthodox method of treatment of wound healing in mice. International Journal of Parapyschology 3(1):5–24

Grad B 1963 A telekinetic effect on plant growth. International Journal of Parapyschology 6(6):473–498

Grad B 1965 Some biological effects of the 'laying on of hands' – a review of experiments with animals and plants. Journal of American Society for Psychical Research 59(1):95–127

Green R 1986 Healing and spirituality. The Practitioner 230:1087–1093

Gribbon J 1989 Quantum rules OK! New Scientist: Inside Science 25 (September 16)

Harrison A 1986 Therapeutic Touch: getting the massage. Nursing Times 82(48):34–35

Haviland D 1986 Safety of faith healing. The Lancet March 22:684

Hawking S J 1988 A brief history of time. Bantam, London

Hayward J 1975 Information: a prescription against pain. Royal College of Nursing, London

Heidt P R 1981 Effects of Therapeutic Touch on anxiety level of hospitalised patients. Nursing Research 30(1):32–37

Heidt P R 1990 Openness: a qualitative analysis of nurses' and patients' experiences of Therapeutic Touch. Image: Journal of Nursing Scholarship 22(3):180–186

Heidt P R 1991 Helping patients to rest: clinical studies in Therapeutic Touch. Holistic Nursing Practice 5(4):57–66

Hodgkinson L 1990 Spiritual healing. Piatkus, London

Hover-Kramer D 1990 Energy fields: implications for the science of caring. Imprint 37(3):7–11

Keller E, Bzdek U M 1986 Effects of Therapeutic Touch on tension headache pain. Nursing Research 2(35):101–105

Krieger D 1975 Therapeutic Touch: the imprimatur of nursing. American Journal of Nursing 5(75):784–787

Krieger D 1979 The Therapeutic Touch: how to use your hands to help or heal. Prentice Hall, New York

Krieger D 1990 Therapeutic Touch. Imprint 37(3):86–88

Krieger D, Ancoli S, Peper E 1979 Searching for evidence of physiological change. American Journal of Nursing 79(4):660–663

Laffan G 1993 A new holistic science. Nursing Standard 7(17):44–45

Liberman R 1962 An analysis of the placebo phenomenon. Journal of Chronic Diseases 15:761–783

Lionberger H 1985 An interpretive study of nurses' practice of Therapeutic Touch. Doctoral Dissertation, University of California, San Francisco

McCorkle R 1974 Effects of touch on seriously ill patients. Nursing Research 23(2):123–125

MacManaway B, Turcan J 1983 Healing: the energy that can restore health. Thorsons, London

MacNutt F 1979 Healing. Bantam, London

Macrae J 1988 Therapeutic Touch: a practical guide. Arkana, London

Malinski V M 1991 Spirituality as integrality: a Rogerian perspective on the path of healing. Journal of Holistic Nursing 9(1):54–64

Meehan T C 1990a Theory development. In: Barrett E A M (ed) Visions of Rogers' science-based nursing. National League for Nursing, New York

Meehan T C 1990b The science of unitary human beings and theory based practice: Therapeutic Touch. In: Barrett E A M (ed) Visions of Rogers' science-based nursing. National League for Nursing, New York

Miller A 1987 Should Christian nurses practice Therapeutic Touch? Journal of Christian Nursing 4(4):15–19

Miller L 1979 An explanation of Therapeutic Touch using the science of unitary man. Nursing Forum 18:278–287

Morse J M, Young D E, Swartz L 1991 Cree Indian healing practices and Western health care: a comparative analysis. Social Science Medicine 32(12):1361–1366

Mulaik J S, Megenity J S, Cannon R B, Gilead M P 1991 Patients' perceptions of nurses' use of touch. Western Journal of Nursing Research 13(3):306–323

Olson M, Sneed N, Bonadonna R, Ratliff J, Dias J 1992 Therapeutic Touch and post-hurricane Hugo stress. Journal of Holistic Nursing 10(2):120–136

Olson M, Sneed N 1995 Anxiety and therapeutic touch. Issues Mental Health Nurse 16:97–108

Olson M, Sneed N, LaVirella G, Bonadonna R, Michel Y 1997 Stress induced immunosuppression and therapeutic touch. Alternative Therapies in Health and Medicine 3(2):68–74

Padmanabhan T 1992 Bridge over the quantum universe. New Scientist 10(37):25–29

Parkes B 1985 Therapeutic Touch as an intervention to reduce anxiety in elderly, hospitalised patients. Doctoral Dissertation, University of Texas, Austin

Payne M B 1989 The use of Therapeutic Touch with rehabilitation clients. Rehabilitation Nursing 14(2)

Peper E, Ancoli S 1976 Two endpoints of an EEG continuum of meditation. In: Krieger D (ed) 1979 The Therapeutic Touch. Prentice Hall, London

Quinn J F 1982 An investigation of the effect of Therapeutic Touch done without physical contact on state anxiety of hospitalised cardiovascular patients. Dissertation Abstracts International 43:1797b

Quinn J F 1984 Therapeutic Touch as energy exchange: testing the theory. Advances in Nursing Science 6(1):42–49

Quinn J F 1988 Building a body of knowledge. Journal of Holistic Nursing 6(1):37–45

Quinn J F 1989a Future directions for Therapeutic Touch research. Journal of Holistic Nursing 7(1):19–25

Quinn J F 1989b Therapeutic Touch as energy exchange: replication and extension. Nursing Science Quarterly 2(2):79–87

Quinn J F 1992 The senior's Therapeutic Touch education programme. Holistic Nursing Practice 7(10):32–37

Randolph G L 1984 Therapeutic Touch and physical touch: physiological response to stressful stimuli. Nursing Research 33(1):33–36

Rogers M E 1970 An introduction to the theoretical basis of nursing. F A Davies, Philadelphia

Rogers M E 1990 Science of unitary human beings. In: Barrett E A M (ed) Visions of Rogers' science-based nursing. National League for Nursing, New York

Sherman J 1985 The laying on of hands. Nursing Times 81(47):18–19

Smith M J 1972 Paranormal effects on enzyme activity. Human Dimensions 1:15–19

Spielberger C D 1970 Anxiety and behaviour. New York. Cited in Heidt P R (1981) Effects of Therapeutic Touch on anxiety level of hospitalised patients. Nursing Research 30(1):32–37

Talbot M 1991 The holographic universe. New York, Harper

Turton P 1988 Healing: therapeutic touch. In Rankin-Box D (ed) Complementary therapies. Chapman Hall, London

Weiss S J 1986 Psychological effects of caregiver touch on incidence of cardiac dysrhythmia. Heart and Lung 15(5):496–503

White J, Krippner S 1977 Future science. Anchor Books, New York

Winstead-Fry P, Kijek J 1999 An integrative review and meta-analysis of Therapeutic Touch research. Alternative Therapies in Health and Medicine 5(6):58–67

Wirth D 1990 The effect of non-contact therapeutic touch on the healing rate of full thickness dermal wounds. Subtle Energies 1(1):1–20

Wirth D, Richardson J T, Eidelman W S, O'Malley A C 1993 Full thickness dermal wounds treated with non-contact therapeutic touch: replication and extension. Complementary Therapies in Health and Medicine 1:127–132

Wirth D, Richardson R, Martinez W, Eidelman W S, Lopez M 1996 Non-contact therapeutic touch intervention and full thickness cutaneous wounds: a replication. Complementary Therapies in Health and Medicine 4:237–240

Wolf S 1950 Effects of suggestion and conditioning on the action of chemical agents in human subjects – the pharmacology of placebos. Journal of Clinical Investigation 29:100–109

Wright S M 1987 The use of Therapeutic Touch in the management of pain. Nursing Clinics of North America 22(3):705–714

Wright S M 1991 Validity of the human energy field assessment form. Western Journal of Nursing Research 13(5):635–648

Zefron L 1975 The history of the laying on of hands. Nursing Forum 15:350–363

SELECTED CASE STUDIES ON THERAPEUTIC TOUCH

Bulbrook M J T 1984 Bulbrook's model of Therapeutic Touch: one form of health and healing in the future. The Canadian Nurse 80(11):30–34

Heidt P R 1991 Therapeutic Touch – the caring environment. Journal of Holistic Nursing 9(3):19–25

Krieger D 1979 The Therapeutic Touch. Prentice-Hall, New York

Macrae J 1979 Therapeutic Touch in practice. American Journal of Nursing 79(4):663–665

3

Providing a conceptual framework for practice

From an original chapter by Francis C Biley, with contributions from Jean Sayre-Adams and Steve Wright

■ *In the deeper reality beyond space and time, we may all be members of one body.*

SIR JAMES JEANS

Roger's Science of Unitary Human Beings

New York University must have been an exciting place to be in the 1960s and 1970s. Dolores Krieger, a Professor in the Division of Nursing, and one-time student of Martha Rogers (Malinski 1993) was beginning to understand and develop TT. At the same time, but as far as can be ascertained from the literature, independently from the work of Dolores Krieger, Martha Rogers, another Professor in the same Division, was beginning to develop what has come to be known as the conceptual framework of the Science of Unitary Human Beings. At the time, and even 30 years on, this provided a radical new vision for nursing and health care. It was unique in offering a framework for practice, education and research that promised a move away from the previously predominant medical model approach to the delivery of nursing and health care. This paradigm shift was happening in other disciplines as well. An enormous rise in interest in and uptake of the use of the complementary therapies was under way – a process still under way today (Foundation for Integrated Medicine 1997). New and often radical approaches to sociology, politics, religion, education, psychology and so on were also coming to the fore at this time, challenging the orthodox views (Friere 1972, Illich 1975 and Rogers 1969, for example).

Martha Rogers' views were a radical alternative to the traditional view of heath care, medicine and nursing, which could be described as Cartesian – that is reductionist, mechanistic and analytic, consisting of 'breaking up thoughts and problems into pieces and arranging these in their logical order' (Capra 1991). Although rooted in nursing, Rogers' work provides us with a helpful framework for the understanding of TT that crosses professional boundaries, and for this reason we include it here for all those interested in TT, regardless of background.

According to some, Rogers' theory has, 'guided nursing out of a concrete, static, closed system world view' (Smith 1989) and, as a result, has challenged many preconceived ideas about nursing and beyond. Indeed, when the theoretical framework was first published, it was, 'in clear contradiction to all the nursing theories in use at that time' (Sarter 1988a). Much of health care in general, and nursing and medicine in particular, had become dominated by reductionist thinking, the application of systems theory and the adoption of task-orientated approaches to health care. Industry had seen the rise of enormous conglomerates and powerful multinationals and the production-line approach to manufacture had been almost universally adopted. So, in health, the emphasis had shifted to technological and therapeutic interventions and controls, breaking down the patient's problems into manageable parts to be taken care of by different carers and therapists.

Rather than just describing nursing as it is, the Science of Unitary Human Beings, which pushed forward (and will continue to push forward), the boundaries of nursing, suggested multiple therapeutic possibilities. It provided a conceptual framework on which to base TT and offered other health disciplines a new perspective for their work. The Science of Unitary Human Beings and Rogerian nursing science offer a view of nursing that is in keeping with current developments in the holistic understanding of the world, such as that suggested by Bohm (1980) and Pribram (1976).

The scale of the influence of the Science of Unitary Human Beings on North American nursing is considerable. Every other year international conferences drawing delegates and presentations from all over the world are held in order to disseminate latest information. The New York-based Society of Rogerian Scholars, which has its members in, for example, North America, Canada, Brazil, Germany and the UK, exists to provide a forum for debate and to enable the exchange of ideas and views through local meetings and the quarterly newsletter the *Rogerian Nursing Science News*. Significant textbooks dedicated to Rogers' work (notably Barrett 1990a, Lutjens 1991, Malinski 1986, Sarter 1988a) have been published. Rogers, up until her death in 1994, was a prolific author and there is a wealth of other published material, with articles frequently appearing in significant nursing journals such as *Nursing Science Quarterly* and *Holistic Nursing Practice*. There is an annual journal entitled *Visions*, containing only work that explores issues raised by the Science of Unitary Human Beings.

Such is the significance of the Rogerian conceptual system that many notable nurse theorists, including for example Rosemary Rizzo

Parse with her theory of 'Human Becoming' and Margaret Newman with her theory of 'Health as Expanding Consciousness', have based their work on the Science of Unitary Human Beings.

The seeds of the conceptual framework, the Science of Unitary Human Beings, were first seen in *Reveille in Nursing*, Rogers' second book, which was published in 1964. Six years later, in 1970, Rogers published an expansion of this earlier work in *An Introduction to the Theoretical Basis of Nursing*. As already stated, there appear to be no explicit, direct links between the developmental work of Dolores Krieger and the formulation of the Science of Unitary Human Beings. However, as will be shown, there are surprising similarities in the proposals suggested by the two nurse academics, and the Science of Unitary Human Beings is now often used as the conceptual framework to support TT (Malinski 1993).

In the 20 years or so that followed the launch of the Science of Unitary Human Beings, considerable changes and developments were made to refine the conceptual framework (Rogers 1980, 1983, 1986, 1990). The original substantive work *An Introduction to the Theoretical Basis of Nursing* is very interesting to read and some would argue that it is a seminal text of historical significance (Lutjens 1991), which in years to come will assume the same importance and significance as Florence Nightingale's *Notes on Nursing*. While it would be an interesting exercise to chart these changes, it is beyond the scope of this chapter, which will give the reader only the most recent currently available definitions of the concepts subsumed under the Science of Unitary Human Beings. At the same time the immense value of these concepts will be emphasised by giving examples of their application in nursing practice and particularly TT, education and research.

The Science of Unitary Human Beings draws on a vast array of subjects that form the theoretical underpinning for the conceptual framework. These include, amongst others, anthropology, astronomy, mathematics (Daily et al 1989), Einsteinian (post-Newtonian) physics (Sarter 1988a) and philosophy, including, amongst others, the work of Polanyi and de Chardin (Sarter 1988b).

It is these origins of the Science of Unitary Human Beings that differentiate the work of Martha Rogers from the work of most other nurse theorists, and also perhaps Dolores Krieger, who developed ideas based on the insights developed from Eastern philosophical thought (Quinn & Strelkauskas 1993). The scope of Rogers' theory also lends itself to study and research in fields of knowledge beyond nursing.

The disciplines Rogers drew from often use terminology in a very specific way and demand an in-depth knowledge and understanding of concepts that are very difficult to express and may be very alien to many of us. It is certainly the reason why it has been called an 'outrageous nursing theory' (Thompson 1990), the complexity of which is 'difficult to understand' (Daily et al 1989) without some knowledge of, for example, quantum physics. However, if an attempt is made to try to understand the conceptual framework (and in some instances this might require prior background reading in some of these supporting subjects), readers will begin to realise why Rogers has been hailed 'a brilliant nurse theorist' and 'one of the most original thinkers in nursing' (Daily et al 1989), without whom it is 'difficult to imagine what nursing would look like today' (Barrett 1990b).

FIVE ASSUMPTIONS

In 1970, Rogers formulated five basic assumptions that describe human beings and their life process (Rogers 1970). These assumptions or 'building blocks', that have more recently been called 'postulates' (Malinski 1993) underpin the conceptual framework and consist of the concepts of:

Wholeness – in which the person is regarded as a unified whole possessing his/her own integrity with characteristics that are more than and different from the sum of the parts. In other words, an individual cannot be divided into, say, a series of systems or 'activities of living' or biological systems such as the nervous, digestive, lymphatic systems and so on. Such an approach is reductionist and fails to address the complexity that makes up the whole person.

Openness – where the individual and the environment are continuously exchanging matter and energy with each other.

Rather than being of solid form, all things are made of energy and only appear solid.

Unidirectionality – where the life process exists along an irreversible space–time continuum. This is a concept that was abandoned in later writings.

Pattern and organisation – which identifies individuals and reflects their innovative wholeness. For example, each person consists of energy that has a particular pattern and organisation and it is this that gives everyone their unique identity.

Sentience and thought – which states that of all life, human beings are the only ones capable of abstraction and imagery, language and thought, sensation and emotion.

FOUR ELEMENTS

In a series of changes that illustrate the ever-developing nature of the Science of Unitary Human Beings over the years since 1970, four 'critical elements' emerged from these basic assumptions that describe the person and the life process (Cowling 1986). These critical elements are now regarded as 'basic to the proposed system' (Rogers 1986) and are:

- energy fields
- open systems
- pattern
- pandimensionality (Rogers 1991).

These four critical elements now form the basis of most of the detailed scientific and philosophical explorations of the Science of Unitary Human Beings and have replaced the previous five building blocks outlined above. They can be described as follows:

Energy fields – the 'fundamental unit of the living and the non-living' (Rogers 1986). They consist of the human energy field and the environment energy field. The human field is, 'an irreducible, indivisible, pandimensional energy field identified by pattern and manifesting characteristics that are specific to the whole and which cannot be predicted from knowledge of the parts' (Rogers 1991). The environmental field is integral with the human field. Each environmental field is specific to its given human field. In other words, 'what has previously been regarded as solid matter now needs to be considered energy with ... the illusion of solidity' (Biley 1993). Although the human field is different from the environment field, they are integral and inseparable, and there can therefore be no exchange of energy between the different fields. It is this aspect of the Science of Unitary Human Beings that does not sit happily with the construction described by Dolores Krieger, who believes that there is an exchange of energy between a field with a healthy abundance of energy and a field of reduced energy that can be utilised when healing (Krieger 1979).

Open systems or openness – describes the open nature of the fields, which allows for a continuous interchange of energy between the fields.

Pattern – the 'distinguishing characteristic of the energy field perceived as a single wave' (Rogers 1986), which gives identity to the field. Human behaviour can be regarded as manifestations of changing pattern (Alligood 1989).

Pandimensionality – describes 'a non-linear domain without special or temporal attributes' (Rogers 1991). It is fundamentally different from the three-dimensional world that we usually view. Pandimensionality (previously known as multidimensionality and prior to that in the early publications, four-dimensionality) is a term that would be used by Rogerian scientists to describe what might otherwise be labelled supernatural experiences or encounters, astral projection, spiritual events, déjà vu and so on.

THREE PRINCIPLES

Such a brief summary of the fundamental basis of the Science of Unitary Human Beings does not do justice to the concepts outlined and does little to explain them. An outline is necessary, however, in order to place in context the key to the conceptual framework, the *Principles of Homeodynamics*. These principles 'postulate a way of perceiving unitary man' (Rogers 1970) and arise from these previous statements, giving 'fundamental guides to the practice of nursing' (Rogers 1990). The *Principles of Homeodynamics* consist of the three principles of:

- integrality

- helicy

- resonancy.

It is these aspects of the Science of Unitary Human Beings that have had more direct relevance for nursing practice, research and education than the descriptions of human beings and the life process that have previously been outlined.

Integrality – describes the 'continuous mutual human field and environmental field process' (Rogers 1990), suggesting that human and environment energy fields are open systems that continuously pass through one another (Alligood 1989).

Helicy – describes the 'continuous innovative, unpredictable, increasing diversity of human and environmental field patterns' (Rogers 1990), the 'continuous creative development and evolution of the human–environmental fields' (Gueldner 1989).

Resonancy – describes the 'continuous change from lower to higher frequency wave patterns in human and environmental fields' (Rogers 1990).

In order to gain a greater understanding of these principles, rather than try to explain the precise way in which these words have been used (a process that is extremely difficult if not impossible), it is probably more useful to see how different authors have interpreted them in their research and practice.

Integrality

The principle of integrality, where the human field is integral or at one with its environmental field (Schodt 1989), was studied by McDonald (1986), who stated that if there is a continuous mutual human field and environmental process, changes in one field will bring about changes in the other. In other words, 'researchers should be able to demonstrate a relationship between a nurse-initiated modi-fication in a person's environment and an alteration in that person's state of being' (McDonald 1986). In order to examine whether such nursing concepts can be brought down the ladder of abstraction to an operational level (Smith 1986), McDonald tested whether an alter-ation in the colour of light (the environmental field) could bring about a reduction in rheumatoid arthritis pain in the left hands of 60 female volunteers (human fields) and found that blue light waves were related to a reduction in the experience of pain. Such findings re-emphasise a whole new world of health care possibilities. It has been suggested that other interventions, such as music (Smith 1986), humour or meditation can be used by the nurse to promote positive human–environment field patterning (Malinski 1986).

Helicy

The principle of helicy was explored by Floyd (1983) who made the prediction that the amount of wakefulness and the number of sleep–wakefulness cycles increase (in other words, there will be an increasing diversity of human and environmental field patterns) when, 'persons experience a deviation in the rhythmic relationship with their environment' (Floyd 1983). Shift rotation and admission to hospital were two variables that were identified as possibly causing diversity in field patterning. Sixty shift workers and 35 hospital in-patients took part in the study, which found that those with diversity in field patterning did indeed sleep less (0.3 hour and 1.0 hour less per cycle for shift workers and hospital inpatients, respectively) than those without such diversity. The number of sleep–wakefulness cycles did not increase for hospital inpatients although it did increase for shift workers. Floyd (1983) indicated that this kind of information may be useful when planning, 'optimum systems for around-the-clock delivery of nursing …'. It also indicated that diversity in human and environmental field patterns occurs for individuals on admission to hospital and that nurses and others should take steps to promote positive human–environmental field re-patterning. In another study that examined the principle of helicy, Rawnsley (1986) found that perceptions of the speed of time were slower for those who were dying and that this could be an explanation for the lack of patience often experienced by the terminally ill.

Resonancy

The principle of resonancy, in which it is suggested that there is a continuous change from lower to higher frequency wave patterns in human and environmental field patterns, has been studied, for example, by Butcher & Parker (1988). These researchers postulated that the technique of guided imagery could promote resonancy, and that the change from lower to higher frequency patterning could be a theoretical explanation for feelings such as relaxation and timelessness. Sixty adult subjects were assigned to an experimental group (who listened to a guided imagery tape) or a control group (who listened to an educational tape). The experimental group had a significantly lower score on the specially developed Time Metaphor Test than the control group, indicating a greater sense of timelessness or higher frequency wave patterning. Subjective opinions from both groups confirmed these results. The authors state that these results illustrate, 'the potential of the Science of Unitary Human Beings for providing a scientific rationale of the use of pleasant guided imagery' (Butcher & Parker 1988), which can promote harmony, relaxation and wellbeing.

It has been stated that Rogers' Science of Unitary Human Beings offers a view that is consistent with the currently prevailing world of holism and ecological concern (Cowling 1986) and in a sense was, perhaps still is, ahead of its time. The above examples of empirical explorations of the principles of homeodynamics show how the Science of Unitary Human Beings can provide the philosophical framework for the development of research studies that influence the development of practice. But there are also other areas where the Science of Unitary Human Beings has had a direct application to practice and education.

Practical applications

Many examples have been given of the direct application of the conceptual framework in nursing practice. Bradley (1987) and Hover-Kramer

(1990) promote the importance of the concept of energy fields and its potential in techniques such as TT. Whelton (1979) presented a comprehensive assessment and care plan based on the Science of Unitary Human Beings. It was shown to be useful in guiding nursing intervention and predicting outcomes in the examples given, that is, the care of a patient with decreased cardiac output, diabetes and hypertension and in the care of another patient with a recurrent meningioma.

Another assessment tool based on Rogerian thinking has been developed by Barrett (1988) who states that nurses need to assess 'pattern manifestation' and to promote 'deliberative mutual patterning' (Barrett 1990c). The nursing care of an adolescent with a 'borderline personality disorder' has been described by Thompson (1990), who used the conceptual framework to describe the interpersonal processes of transference and countertransference that existed.

Further explorations of patient care scenarios using the Science of Unitary Human Beings are given by Meehan (1990a), who describes caring for a man with pain due to metastatic cancer, and Madrid (1990), who gives a moving account of successful deliberative mutual patterning in the care of a patient who was in considerable discomfort due to pain, hospitalisation and gastrointestinal bleeding.

Therapeutic Touch and Rogers' Science

In recent years, the Science of Unitary Human Beings has proved to be a relevant framework for the exploration and explanation of TT. Several TT practitioners and theorists, such as Quinn (1984) and Meehan (1990b), have used the Science of Unitary Human Beings as a means of providing a rationale and an explanation for the practice of TT and the foundation for most of the TT studies (Quinn & Strelkauskas 1993). Although this work is regarded as very influential, it has not been without its difficulties and is only in the very early stages of development and understanding.

As already stated, Krieger developed TT on a basis taken from Eastern philosophies and systems of medicine. Energy, or alternatively prana or ch'i, is thought by Krieger to flow from the healthy TT practitioner, who has an abundance, to the ill person with depleted levels of energy. Meehan (1990b) suggested that this concept is incompatible with the Science of Unitary Human Beings, where there is never any, 'to–from exchange or interaction between practitioner and client' (Malinski 1993).

Quinn has therefore re-conceptualised TT and, rather than using a pure Krieger–Kunz method and rationale, has begun to explore what has become known as the Rogerian–Quinn framework for TT (Olson et al 1992).

Meehan (1990b) re-defined TT, 'as a knowledgeable and purposive patterning of patient–environment energy field process in which the nurse assumes a meditative awareness and uses her/his hands as a focus for the patterning of the mutual patient–environment energy field process', suggesting that the Krieger term 'energy exchange' should be changed to the Rogerian term 'energy process' and that 'energy transfer' should become 'mutual process'. She also stated that TT should not be seen as derived from 'laying on of hands'.

Other differences between TT as perceived from a Krieger–Kunz perspective and as perceived from a Science of Unitary Human Beings perspective have been identified (Malinski 1993). Some of these differences are, for example, that from a Rogerian perspective, TT is not seen as a practitioner–patient interaction because the practitioner should be regarded as being part of the patient's environment. It is therefore a practitioner–environment process. Additionally, Rogers prefers to employ words such as participation rather than motivation or intentionality because the, 'Therapeutic Touch practitioner is neither an instrument of nor a conduit for a higher healing power' (Malinski 1993). As was suggested in Chapter 1, perceptions of energy moving, of some higher power intervening and so on may be just that – perceptions, the products of the rational mind as it seeks to bring meaning and clarity to a process which may be altogether ineffable and mysterious (and may remain so). Rogers, in her many writings and speeches, while seeking understanding, always seems to be comfortable with the essential mystery of that which she sought to describe. She was always inclined to encourage those who worked with her ideas to pursue knowledge, and at the same time to feel relaxed and comfortable with the unknown.

Certainly, many TT practitioners report that Rogers gives them a useful framework to explore their practice and gain some idea of what is taking place. It embraces the essential concepts of a holistic approach and holistic theory. In being descriptive, it avoids dogma and is religion neutral, making it adaptable to many perspectives on TT yet providing a reasoned framework and language to examine, explore and explain practice. Even so, TT practitioners report that this is all it can do. The experience of TT transcends any model or theory as we deepen our knowledge and practice of it. Rogers' work provides us with a platform for understanding and illumination of TT, and is especially helpful in giving structure for some who wish to learn about the practice, especially in the early stages.

This exploration of the Science of Unitary Human Beings and the re-conceptualisation of TT is by no means fully comprehensive (more extensive reviews, primarily of the Science of Unitary Human Beings, can be found in Barrett 1990a and Daily et al 1989). Nevertheless, the aforementioned literature provides evidence that points to the expanding adoption of the Science of Unitary Human Beings as a framework to guide the practice of TT in both the relative present and the relative future. Even so, a considerable amount of work needs to be done before a complete reconceptualisation of TT is achieved.

As this chapter has shown, trying to describe the Science of Unitary Human Beings without moving too far away from (and perhaps therefore losing the essential meaning of) the terminology employed by Martha Rogers and other Rogerian scientists is a very difficult task. An understanding of the Science of Unitary Human Beings requires a broadly based unitary knowledge base and education.

Rogers stated that, 'education is for the future, yesterday's methods will not suffice for tomorrow's needs' (Rogers 1961). Rogers' framework provides us with an approach to meet these new educational challenges for health care practitioners in a world of radically altering perspectives on what it is to be healthy, not just for persons, but for communities and the whole planet.

PRACTICAL NOTE

For those interested, examples of Rogerian-based care plans can be found in Biley (1993) and Madrid (1990). Further information on

Rogerian Nursing Science and the Society of Rogerian Scholars can be obtained from: Francis C Biley, School of Nursing Studies, University of Wales College of Medicine, Heath Park, Cardiff, Wales, UK. Tel: 02920 743734.

References

Alligood M R 1989 Rogers' theory and nursing administration: a perspective on health and environment. In: Henry B, Arndt C, DiVincenti M et al (eds) Dimensions of nursing administration: theory, research, education and practice. Blackwell Scientific, Boston

Barrett E A M 1988 Using Rogers' science of unitary human beings in nursing practice. Nursing Science Quarterly 1:50–51

Barrett E A M 1990a Visions of Rogers' science-based nursing. National League for Nursing, New York

Barrett E A M 1990b Preface. In: Barrett E A M (ed) Visions of Rogers' science-based nursing. National League for Nursing, New York

Barrett E A M 1990c Rogers' science-based nursing practice. In: Barrett E A M (ed) Visions of Rogers' science-based nursing. National League for Nursing, New York

Biley F C 1993 Energy fields nursing: a brief encounter of a unitary kind. International Journal of Nursing Studies 30(6):519–525

Bohm D 1980 Wholeness and the implicate order. Routledge, London

Bradley D B 1987 Energy fields: implications for nurses. Journal of Holistic Nursing 5(11): 32–35

Butcher H K, Parker N I 1988 Guided imagery within Rogers' science of unitary human beings: an experimental study. Nursing Science Quarterly 1:103–110

Capra F 1991 The Tao of Physics. Shambhala, Boston

Cowling W R 1986 The science of unitary human beings: theoretical issues, methodological challenges, and research realities. In: Malinski V M (ed) Explorations on Martha Rogers' science of unitary human beings. Appleton-Century-Croft, Connecticut

Daily J S, Maupin J S, Slattery M C, Schmell D L, Wallace T L 1989 Martha E Rogers: unitary human beings. In: Marriner-Tomey A (ed) Nursing theorists and their work, 2nd edn. Mosby, New York

Floyd J A 1983 Research using Rogers' conceptual system: development of a testable theorem. Advances in Nursing Science 5(2):37–48

Foundation for Integrated Medicine 1997 Integrated Healthcare. FIM, London.

Freire P 1972 Pedagogy of the oppressed. Penguin, Harmondsworth.

Gueldner S H 1989 Applying Rogers' model to nursing administration: emphasis on client and nursing. In: Henry B, Arndt C, DiVincenti M, Marriner-Tomey A (eds) Dimensions of nursing administration: theory, research, education and practice. Blackwell Scientific, Boston

Hover-Kramer D 1990 Energy fields: implications for the science of human caring. Imprint 37(3):81–82

Krieger D 1979 The therapeutic touch: how to use your hands to help or heal. Prentice-Hall, New Jersey

Illich I 1975 Medical nemesis. Penguin, Harmondsworth

Lutjens L R J 1991 Martha E Rogers: the science of unitary human beings. Sage, London

McDonald S F 1986 The relationship between visible lightwaves and the experience of pain. In: Malinski V M (ed) Explorations on Martha E Rogers' science of unitary human beings. Appleton-Century-Crofts, Connecticut

Madrid M 1990 The participating process of human field patterning in an acute-care environment. In: Barrett E A M (ed) Visions of Rogers' science-based nursing. National League for Nursing, New York

Malinski V M 1986 Explorations on Martha E Rogers' science of unitary human beings. Appleton-Century-Crofts, Connecticut

Malinski V M 1993 Therapeutic touch: the view from Rogerian nursing science. Visions 1(1):45–54

Meehan T C 1990a The science of unitary human beings and theory based practice: Therapeutic Touch. In: Barrett E A M (ed) Visions of Rogers' science-based nursing. National League for Nursing, New York

Meehan T C 1990b Theory development. In: Barrett E A M (ed) Visions of Rogers' science-based nursing. National League for Nursing, New York

Olson M, Sneed N, Bonadonna R, Ratcliff J, Dias 1992 Therapeutic Touch and post-hurricane Hugo stress. Journal of Holistic Nursing 10:120–136

Pribram K H 1976 Problems concerning the structure of consciousness. In: Globus G (ed) Consciousness and the brain. Plenum, New York

Quinn J F 1984 Therapeutic Touch as energy exchange: testing the theory. Advances in Nursing Science 6(2):42–49

Quinn J F, Strelkauskas A J (1993) Psychoimmunologic effects of Therapeutic Touch on practitioners and recently bereaved recipients: a pilot study. Advances in Nursing Science 15(4):13–26

Rawnsley M M 1986 The relationship between the perception of the speed of time and the process of dying. In: Malinski V M (ed) Explorations on Martha Rogers' science of unitary human beings. Appleton-Century-Crofts, Connecticut

Rogers C 1969 Freedom to learn. F A Davis, Philadelphia

Rogers M E 1961 Educational revolution in nursing. Macmillan, New York

Rogers M E 1964 Reveille in nursing. F A Davis, Philadelphia

Rogers M E 1970 An introduction to the theoretical basis of nursing. F A Davis, Philadelphia

Rogers M E 1980 Nursing: a science of unitary man. In: Riehl J P and Roy C (eds) Conceptual models for nursing practice, 2nd edn. Appleton-Century-Crofts, New York

Rogers M E 1983 Science of unitary human beings: a paradigm for nursing. In: Clements I W, Roberts F B (eds) Family health: a theoretical approach to nursing care. Wiley, New York

Rogers M E 1986 Science of unitary human beings. In: Malinski V M (ed) Explorations on Martha Rogers' science of unitary human beings. National League for Nursing, New York

Rogers M E 1990 Nursing: science of unitary, irreducible, human beings: update 1990. In: Barrett E A M (ed) Visions of Rogers' science-based nursing. National League for Nursing, New York

Rogers M E 1991 Glossary. Rogerian Nursing Science News 4(2):6–7

Sarter B 1988a The stream of becoming: a study of Martha Rogers' Theory. National League for Nursing, New York

Sarter B 1988b Philosophical sources of nursing theory. Nursing Science Quarterly 1:32–59

Schodt C M 1989 Parental–fetal attachment and couvade: a study of patterns of human–environment integrality. Nursing Science Quarterly 2(2):88–97

Smith M J 1986 Human–environment process: a test of Rogers' principle of integrality. Advances in Nursing Science 9(1):21–28

Smith M J 1989 Four dimensionality: where to go with it. Nursing Science Quarterly 2(2):56

Thompson J E 1990 Finding the borderline's border: can Martha Rogers help? Perspectives in Psychiatric Care 26(4):7–10

Whelton B J 1979 An operationalisation of Martha Rogers' theory throughout the nursing process. International Journal of Nursing Studies 16:7–20

4

The essentials of practice

Jean Sayre-Adams   Steve Wright

Explorations
Several steps
Related issues
Factors affecting success

■ *'I can't believe that' said Alice.*

■ *'Can't you?' the Queen wailed in a pitying tone.*

■ *'Try again; draw a long breath, and shut your eyes.'*

LEWIS CARROLL   *Through the Looking Glass*

This chapter will suggest some experiential exercises and give some case studies as well as address some of the questions that are most asked about TT. It is important, however, that anyone reading this book recognises from the outset that the safe practice of TT cannot be learned from books. We strongly recommend anyone wishing to practice TT to pursue a recognised course of study, some suggestions for which will be given in the last chapter.

Explorations

This exercise was devised by Krieger (1979) and is now widely used.

EXERCISE 1 THERAPEUTIC TOUCH SELF-KNOWLEDGE TEST

1. Bring your attention to your hands (Fig. 4.1). You may perhaps explore one hand with the other. Stretch and wiggle the fingers and wrists. Perhaps you may want to rub your palms together. Become more aware of your hands and how they serve you.

2. Then sit comfortably with both feet on the ground and simply place your hands so that the palms face each other (Fig. 4.2). Hold your elbows away from the trunk of your body and do not rest your lower arms in your lap. Now bring your palms as close together as you can without having them touch each other, so that they are perhaps one-eighth to one-quarter of an inch apart.

3. Separate the palms of your hands by about 2 inches and then slowly bring them back to their original position.

4. Now separate your palms by about 4 inches and, again, slowly bring them back to their original position.

5. Repeat this procedure. However, this time, separate your palms by about 6 inches. Keep your motions slow and steady. As you return your hands to their original position, notice any sensations you begin to feel in, around and between your hands. You may feel pressure, heat, tingling, etc.

Figure 4.1 *'Bring your attention to your hands'.*

Figure 4.2 *Exercise 1.*

6. Once again separate your palms, this time until they are about 8 inches apart. Do not immediately return your hands to their original position. Instead, as you bring your hands close together, notice what you experience as you try stopping for a moment every 2 inches or so. What sensations do you experience? Perhaps tingling, pressure, pulling and so on? It is particularly important to stay relaxed and centred in this exercise, just paying attention to what is happening in and around your hands. Everyone's experiences will be different, but reports of pressure between the hands, of a 'bouncy' feeling, extremes of heat or cold, stickiness, a magnetic 'pulling' feeling between the hands – all of these and more are common.

7. Spend the next full minute in experiencing this field between your hands and try to determine what other characteristics of the field you feel besides those already noted.

No one to date has been able to measure the exchange of 'energy'. However, people who have had what they perceive as the experience of this energy exchange (either by feeling or sometimes seeing energy fields) have no doubt of its existence.

The following incident leaves us with even more questions:

We had finished the first day of a two-day introductory TT workshop with an experience and discussion about energy fields and the colours yellow, orange and red. Leaving all that behind, another of the participants and I went to pick her children up from school. We moved into talking with the children about their day and continued after we got home, focusing on the children's issues, not thinking or talking about the TT class at all. One of the girls disappeared for half an hour and when she returned she brought with her a picture which she showed to me. I asked her who it was, and she told me it was me. I commented on how pretty I appeared to her and then asked her what the lines around me were. She told me that it was my 'pattern' and that my pattern looked pretty to her when it was that colour.

Several steps

Almost every article on TT lists four, five or six steps on how to perform TT. It should be emphasised that while most teachers do use a step-by-step method when actually teaching TT, these steps are not sequential, nor necessarily done in a linear fashion. They flow into one another and it is often impossible for someone watching to distinguish one step from another. Thus we use the terms 'steps' or 'phases' here to help the student of TT to gain an understanding of what is taking place in the initial stages. The experienced practitioner will soon learn that the practice of TT goes beyond these initial descriptions.

Figure 4.3 *Humans are not the only ones to respond to TT.*

CENTRING

Centring is achieved by shifting awareness from an external to an internal focus, becoming relaxed and calm and making a mental intention to assist the patient.

Lionberger (1985) describes centring as 'a method for:

1. disciplining attention

2. achieving calm

3. establishing receptivity'.

Centring is focusing on the here and now, placing oneself in a calm, alert, open state. It involves having a clear sense of oneself as a unitary whole and differs from concentration or paying attention in that it is not associated with mental effort. It brings those who intend to participate in the process into harmony with one another and so mobilises the TT process. Centring is paramount to proceeding with the remaining phases and is necessary for the intervention to be effective. Being unable to become or stay centred causes the practitioner to feel depleted of energy and tired, and they become ineffectual (Sayre-Adams 1993). Many people experience a state of expanded consciousness when they centre.

In the practice of TT, we are always attentive to the holistic nature of healing. That which affects ourselves, the environment and those seeking healing is all caught up in an interacting world. What we bring to this process contributes to the whole. If our consciousness is disturbed, if we are unwell, ill at ease or unhappy, we may find that this affects the person we seek to help as well. If we are not fully centred, then we are more likely to experience negative effects as a result of practising TT with someone. Students often use the words 'calm', 'peaceful', 'integrated', 'aligned', 'grounded', 'whole', 'at one' and 'in harmony with their environment' to describe how they feel when they are centred. The words used are almost as varied as the number of students. Equally as varied are the ways in which different practitioners arrive at their centre. Many find that a meditation practice is helpful in learning to centre quickly and to stay centred (see the section on meditation on p. 108).

EXERCISE 2 **A CENTRING TECHNIQUE**

If you have not found your own way of centring yet, you could try the exercise below. It has been used in TT classes for many years.

1. Sit comfortably and close your eyes.

2. Inhale and exhale deeply.

3. Focus your mind on some image in nature, such as a tree or a mountain, which brings you a sense of peace. If you become distracted, gently bring your mind back to your image of peace. Remember not to tighten up or try to force your mind to be still. Just maintain a calm but firm intent to keep focused on the image.

ASSESSMENT

Whether working in hospitals, clinics, private offices or on the streets, health care professionals use their assessment skills from the first contact. In hospitals, they look at X-rays, laboratory results, vital signs, skin tone, skin colour and so on. In some specialist units each system may be assessed, e.g. cardiac, respiratory, neurological. When working in places other than hospitals, the assessment may be to observe the walking/movement, tone of voice, grooming or body language.

The assessment of the pattern or energy field (in Rogerian terms) or, to put it more simply, what we feel with our hands and intuition about that person (just as we 'felt' things in our hands in Exercise 1 at the start of this chapter) is what determines the next stage of our practice. It is not a diagnostic tool. The imbalances and other things that we may experience as we assess do not necessarily indicate some underlying pathology. We may feel heat, for example, in the area above an inflamed knee, but a tingling sensation perceived around the head does not necessarily indicate a brain tumour, nor does a heavy or sticky sensation felt around the abdomen indicate bowel disease. We have to remember that what we are experiencing here is the effect of two unique people/energy patterns coming together, at least one of whom is paying close attention to the other with conscious, healing intention. Thus what we experience in assessment may or may not correspond to the symptoms of the patient according to any medical diagnosis they may have. In one sense it matters little, because we are not seeking 'cures' here, we are seeking healing (see Chapter 1), and healing may or may not be linked to a person's obvious health problem.

The person carrying out the assessment needs to be relaxed, with their mind open, and centred. The assessment is done by holding the hands 3 to 5 inches from the physical body of the person and moving them along and over the length of the body/energy field from head to toe, checking for 'imbalances' or differences in the field. There can be many variations in what we experience. Furthermore, one practitioner is unlikely to have the same experience as another, for each of us brings our unique qualities/pattern to the healing relationship, and that pattern may be shifting from moment to moment. This of course brings major challenges for researchers because so many variables are at work. It is simply not possible for one practitioner to check the assessment of another and hope to get the same 'results', for the impact of the first interaction with the first practitioner and even a short moment of time may have affected the pattern that can be felt by the next practitioner – who in turn brings their own unique interaction to bear.

Practitioners report that a balanced field might have a 'soft', 'rhythmic', 'even' or 'warm' feel. Imbalances are highly subjective and will be perceived as subtly as the feeling in the hands in the TT self-knowledge test (Exercise 1). Some of the words used by students to describe these imbalances are 'warmth', 'cold', 'pins and needles', 'void', 'empty', 'heavy' and 'pressure'. More experienced practitioners also perceive information through intuitive and somatic clues rather than through the hands, although the hands still seem to be the focal point for these clues. For example, the person practising TT may simply feel that they 'know' where the imbalance in the energy field is. Or they may feel it in a corresponding place in their own body, e.g. a patient's headache may be experienced as a pain in the head of the practitioner.

Figure 4.4 *Assessing.*

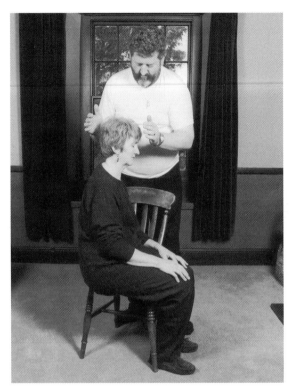

Figure 4.5 *Therapeutic Touch-using the hands to help and heal.*

I find now that when working with patients I seem no longer to be as focused on sensations around their bodies. This was something I learned in the early stages and relied upon very much. Now I get a sense of 'knowing' things. Often I can 'see' something in my mind's eye that the patient upon questioning reports that they are thinking about. Sometimes I get impressions of some old or hurtful memory that seems to fit with something they want to explore with me. Sometimes it is insights into their past, people they have loved or who have loved them and so on. I have to work quite hard not to get too attached to the phenomena, but to accept them as they are, to work with the patients to see what meaning it has for them.

TT practitioner with 10 years experience

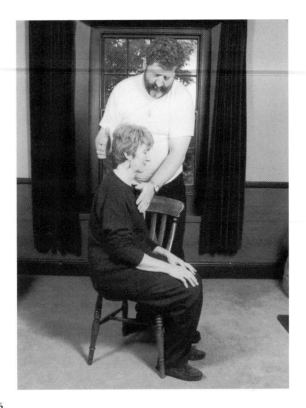

Figure 4.6

Krieger (1993) has found that most often the imbalances that are picked up in the assessment phase are one or a combination of the following.

- temperature differentials, such as a sense of heat or cold

- pressure or feelings of congestion in the energy flow

- changes in or lack of synchronisation in the intrinsic rhythmicity of the patient's energy field

- localised weak electric shocks or tingly feelings.

The clues are qualitative and difficult to describe precisely. Because assessing is always an ongoing process, it should not be a cause of concern if all the cues are not picked up the first time. Assessment and treatment of the patient may be carried out in any position he or she feels comfortable with. The following tips are given to ensure a successful assessment:

EXERCISE 3 SUGGESTIONS FOR THE ASSESSMENT

Below are step-by-step suggestions for the assessment. Either try these or develop your own.

The following suggestion is taken from the work of Macrae (1987):

1. Ask the patient to sit on a stool or sideways on a chair so that his/her back is unobstructed.

2. Sit, kneel or stand to the side of the patient so that one of your hands – either the right or the left – extends in front of the patient and the other is behind the patient's back.

3. Pass your hands gently through the patient's energy field (about 3 to 5 inches from the surface of the skin), palms facing the body, starting from the top of the head and moving down to the feet. When the hand at the back reaches the patient's hips, keep it there while the other hand passes all the way down the legs to the feet.

or:

1. Ask the patient to sit on a stool or sideways on a chair.

2. Sit, kneel or stand in front of the patient; then pass your hands, parallel to each other with palms facing the patient, through the patient's energy field from head to foot.

3. Assess the back of the patient and pass your hands, in the same manner, from the patient's head down to the hips.

More tips:

1. Make all your movements down from top to bottom.

2. Your complete assessment should not exceed 60–90 seconds.

3. Do not linger on a spot while trying to decide what you feel. If in doubt, repeat the whole assessment again (starting with

centring) from the beginning to ascertain the correctness of your cues.

4. If you lose your centre, stop, recentre yourself and start from the beginning.

5. Feel the arches of the feet to see if the 'energy' coming from them is equal, i.e. the pattern you sense is balanced and harmonious, smooth and even. If not, clear the blockage before you go any further (see next step).

6. Do not try too hard. This is an intuitive process and should be allowed to unfold.

CLEARING

In this step (Fig 4.7), the hands are used to facilitate a sense of a symmetrical and rhythmical flow of energy through the field. In other words, the intention is to facilitate a sense of smoothness and even-ness, comfort and balance across the whole of the patient's body. It is done by sweeping the hands just above the body, downward. The entire body is covered, with concentration over the areas where an imbalance or blockage was identified during the assessment.

In Krieger's (1979) view, it is in this phase that the patients mobilise their own resources so that self-healing can occur. It is commonly reported that responses indicative of deep relaxation occur most frequently during this phase. If the patient is experiencing anxiety, discomfort or pain of a physical or emotional nature, it is at this point that these symptoms may diminish. A visible or audible relaxation response from the patient, e.g. a deep breath or sigh, peripheral flush, deepening of the voice or other signs of physical relaxation, perhaps even sleep, will often be observed. Many practitioners believe this is not a separate step but part of the balancing or repatterning phase. Certainly the assessment, clearing and repatterning are performed concurrently and repetitively.

The act of clearing frees any sense of blockage or imbalance in the patient's field. A sense of energy being unblocked is achieved. It can also be used to:

Figure 4.7 *Clearing.*

- facilitate energy flow

- break up energy patterns, such as congestion

- re-establish rhythm in the patient's energy field

- cool, in situations such as elevated temperature

- move patterned energy within the field

- knit together the energy field.

It is intentionality, not hand movement, which is important (Krieger 1993). Once again the use of terms from Rogerian and post-Einsteinian thinking is offered with caution. They help in some degree to describe what is taking place. Practitioners can assert that they 'feel' something, but whether it is strictly 'energy' or 'fields' is open to debate. Certainly these concepts and experiences fit well within Rogerian theory, and give us a framework that seeks to describe what is taking place.

TREATMENT – BALANCING OR REPATTERNING

Once a sense of symmetrical flow of energy has been facilitated in the energy field through clearing, then the practitioner returns to the places where the imbalances were felt in the assessment and repatterns the field using intention and clear visualisation (Fig 4.8). For instance, if the imbalance were perceived as cold, the practitioner would seek to envision it warming and vice versa. If a pressure was felt, an attempt would be made to reduce that pressure; if congestion, an attempt would be made to loosen and remove that congestion and so on. These changes or repatterning are accomplished through the appropriate direction, modulation or guidance of energy from one area of the energy field of the patient to another or from the environmental field to the patient.

During this phase, as in all others, the practitioner continues to sense their own field continually, simultaneously and mutually as a part of the patient's field, as well as the environmental field. Ultimately, there is really no distinction when fields are intact.

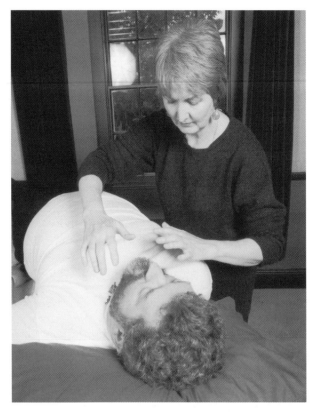

Figure 4.8 *Repatterning*

Intentions that you may have for the repatterning phase may be as follows:

- facilitation of the energy flow
- stimulation of the energy flow
- mobilisation of congestion or pressure in the energy field
- dampening or quieting of energetic activity
- synchronisation of rhythmicity in the energy flow.

Although these phases are usually taught sequentially to beginners, with experienced practitioners they become more dynamic and

Mike had been with me for weekly TT sessions for over 10 weeks. He had chronic psoriasis, with involvement of some joints, and a long history of mental health and social problems. He had been referred to me as one of those 'hopeless' cases who didn't seem to respond to anyone's efforts (over decades) – passed from physician, to nurse, to social worker, to psychiatrist, etc. Each person had tried to tackle some or all of his problems to little avail. His situation was compounded by an unsettled home life in a poor area of the city, dependency on drugs, unemployment, alcoholism, a difficult and sometimes abusive relationship with his now deceased father – in fact this man seemed to have just about every problem that life could throw at him.

The most immediate impact on him was a deep relaxation response, and at each session he began to talk about his feelings and many issues that affected him deeply. Often, I would find myself sensing his disturbed state when he walked in the room, though to all intents and purposes he seemed quite stable. Sometimes, I just knew things were going badly for him sometimes hours or days before we would meet again. Sometimes during a session I would have visual experiences that seemed to coincide with what he was experiencing. For example, we would regularly have conversations like this:

Me: 'Tell me what you are thinking now, Mike'.
Mike: 'I was just thinking about my dog and the walks we used to have.'
Me: 'That's interesting, I'm getting the same image.'

I'm not at all sure what was taking place, but this sort of synchronicity was extremely common with this, and other patients as my practice deepened. I learned to use these insights with Mike and others in careful ways. Sometimes taking him on imaginary journeys with his dog, for example, from which he gained insights himself about his relationships, why he got angry and how to deal with it and so on. As the weeks went by he was able, at his request, to come off all his antidepressants and antipsychotics, came off the drink, his psoriasis was less inflamed, he took steps to get a job, learned how not to get caught up in the family fights, and came to a place of forgiveness for his father and so on. What was happening with him, and the courage with which he pursued many difficult things profoundly impressed me.

Cont'd

He saw it all as 'down to me' so I had to watch this – how easily I could get caught in the 'great healer' trap, how I had to gently coach him in words he could understand to accept that this was mutual work, and not one sided.

At the time, the talk in the health services was all about 'evidence-based medicine'. I thought, how do I fit this one in? There wasn't that much change in his physical condition, that could hardly be put down to TT, and there were so many other variables, other treatments and practitioners of all sorts you would have been hard pushed to say that TT did anything at all. Also, with so much emphasis on the physical state as his health problem, feeling better about himself, being less angry and things like that didn't seem to count for much in the way treatments are evaluated. What I do know is that his experience with me in TT was like nothing else he had experienced with any other carer, that he significantly moved on in the way he was in the world (for the better in his and everyone else's view) and all this after 25 years of seemingly intractable social and health problems. Something had worked for him, and it was beyond any perceptions of energy fields or patterns. My practice seemed to have moved to a deep, trusting and wondrous place that I find it difficult to describe, but where I was privileged to witness healing for this man emerge.

TT practitioner with 10 years experience

are often performed concurrently and repetitively. It is often difficult for an observer to notice distinct phases (Sayre-Adams 1994).

EVALUATION

A treatment can last anything from a few seconds to half an hour or more, and is 'finished' when the sense of repatterning or rebalancing is complete. This is perceived intuitively by experienced practitioners or when a reassessment shows that balancing is achieved. A shorter time will always be needed when working with babies, frail or debilitated patients and when applying TT to the head area. Pregnant women, patients in shock and patients with mental health problems are also often more sensitive.

This summary of treatment is revised from Macrae (1987):

1. Do your preliminary relaxation and centring exercise. Feel your energy field becoming at one with the energy field of your patient and the rest of the environment.

2. Place your intent upon the wholeness and wellbeing of the patient.

3. Gently massage the patient's neck and shoulders.

4. When you are centred and the patient is relaxed, assess the quality of their energy field.

5. Clear away any loose congestion (thickness, heat, pressure), making sure that the energy is flowing freely through the feet.

6. Loosen any obstructions (cold or blank areas) so that the field is open and flowing.

7. Fill in depleted areas, where you feel a pulling sensation.

8. Stop immediately and recentre yourself if you become drained of your own energy or if you absorb the patient's pain or problems.

9. Reassess the energy field of the patient from time to time and clear away any congestion that may have surfaced.

10. Observe the patient for signs of relaxation (e.g. slower and deeper breathing, flushed face, muscle twitching).

11. If appropriate, ask for feedback from the patient and modify the treatment accordingly.

12. Conclude the treatment when the deficits have been filled in and the energy field is flowing in an open, even manner.

13. Ask the patient to sit or lie quietly for 20–30 minutes. These steps are not always performed sequentially. The more experienced the practitioner, the more these steps become one continuous, flowing movement.

When I first met Mr J, a 61-year-old farmer, and invited him to come into the treatment room, I thought I would have to stop him falling over. His gait was unsteady but he did not require assistance.

Mr J told me that over the last 15 years his balance had progressively deteriorated to such an extent that, with very few exceptions, he fell every day. Some of the falls had resulted in a broken nose and arm, and cuts and bruises of varying severity. He said that many people thought he was drunk and his walk certainly gave that impression. He stated that his problems were due to a hereditary disease, that he was not receiving any medication and that his doctors were unable to do anything to help him.

Before commencing with TT, I centred myself by visualising an oak tree with its leaves shimmering in a gentle breeze and inwardly calming myself by taking a few deep breaths. I visualised a universal power of which I became a part. This personal method of centring is one which I find effective.

With Mr J lying on his back, I began TT. His initial assessment revealed on overall feeling of coolness in his energy field. As I had not felt any particular energy block or areas of deficit, my intuition led me to gently move towards Mr J's abdominal area and start the rebalancing. I imagined a warm soothing light encompassing Mr J. I again moved my hands in a head-to-toe direction to reassess and continued and rebalancing, moving my hands in a continuous, flowing manner. I continued this for approximately 10 minutes, until a feeling of warmth replaced the coolness. The same feeling of coolness was felt down the spinal column. This too was replaced with warmth after the rebalancing or repatterning.

Mr J had had no sensations but said 'inwardly something is happening' and 'is it possible to feel better immediately?' His gait was unchanged.

The following week, the returned and was over the moon with how well he felt. He called me the lady with the oilcan – his joints were no longer stiff and he had not fallen all week. He was able to negotiate the steps in his house without having to hold onto the door frame and he could put his shoes on without having to sit down.

On the second and third visits there were still areas of coolness in the energy fields around his legs and spinal column, or static-type shocks. A repatterning was down on the third visit and Mr J experienced a 'sensation travelling down my body.'

Three weeks later, he had his fourth and final TT treatment. At this time his energy field felt complete and he had not fallen fox 6 weeks. His unsteady gait was still evident, but was not as exaggerated and he felt better able to cope. I believe TT improved Mr J's quality of life, enhanced his feeling of wellbeing and reduced his risk of physical injury through falls.

Related issues

MEDITATION

Meditation is often misunderstood. Perhaps this is because there are so many ways to meditate. The purpose of meditation is simply to develop a sense of awareness, focus intentionality (see p. 113), insight and a selfless attitude. Meditation allows people to uncover, recover and discover parts of themselves of which they have not previously been aware. Meditation can be a bridge between the inner and outer worlds.

There are a great many types of meditation – lying down meditations, sitting meditations, standing meditations, walking meditations. There are breath meditations, sound meditations, visual meditations. Some are achieved through the intellect (most popular in our Western society), through the emotions (used most frequently by mystics), through the body (as in yoga or dancing), or through action (as in concentrating on a particular skill such as rug making or perhaps gardening) to make it perfect. There are structured meditations and unstructured meditations. TT is sometimes called a healing meditation. This was because when subjects were attached to EEG machines, the EEG of the 'meditator' and TT practitioner were similar (Peper & Ancoli 1976).

EXERCISE 4 **INTRODUCTION TO MEDITATION**

You might wish to try different kinds of meditation until you find one that suits you. Whatever your choice, you should feel better for it. Try it for 10 or 15 minutes a day to begin with. Many books, tapes and so on are available as guides to different techniques. We feel one of the best books on meditation is by Le Shan (1974).

Below is a short, simple meditation you could try out. Before you begin, make sure that you won't be disturbed – use a quiet place where you will not be interrupted by others, telephone calls, etc.

1. Sit quietly, feet on the floor, eyes closed.

2. Become aware of your breathing.

3. Breathe slowly in and out, counting each time you breathe in, until you have counted up to four breaths, then continue to count the breaths from one to four.

4. Just be aware of the counting – as fully aware as possible.

5. When your mind wanders or sensations or emotions arise, bring your attention back to the counting.

The goal is to have your whole being involved in the counting.

Try this meditation again with eyes open and add 'and' to each count as you breathe out, i.e. one-and, two-and, three-and, four-and, one-and, and so on. These are only variations.

Start out with 10 or 15 minutes a day. Set your alarm clock so you don't have to look at your watch. You might want to put the clock under a pillow.

HEALTH PROBLEMS RESPONSIVE TO TT

Research has shown that TT can accelerate wound healing, induce physiological relaxation, decrease anxiety, decrease pain, decrease diastolic blood pressure, and reduce stress in hospitalised patients (see Chapters 1 and 2). Clinical practice has shown TT to be particularly useful for upper respiratory tract infections, allergies, headaches and musculoskeletal conditions, as well as being effective on an emotional and sometimes spiritual level. It is extremely useful for promoting comfort for those who are dying. Those who practice TT do not necessarily expect a 'cure' but often see a healing occur.

There are some patients/clients with whom it is wise to proceed with caution and limit your time. These are the frail, pregnant women, babies, people with head injuries, emaciated people (AIDS or cancer patients) and patients with mental health problems. This is not to say that TT is ruled out, rather to emphasise the need to be especially aware and sensitive during the interaction.

TT WITH FAMILY MEMBERS

TT requires the practitioner to be objective and in a place of non-attached compassion. Being objective is sometimes hard with family members or good friends, and it is often difficult to remain centred enough to be effective with them. However, it seems a shame that something so helpful cannot be shared with those we love most. So give it a try! It will be excellent practice for staying objective and centred. Remember, though, if they are very ill and you are upset, it may only add to their discomfort.

TWO PRACTITIONERS WORKING TOGETHER

If two practitioners are available (Fig 4.9), it is both pleasant and effective to work together on the same patient. In this case, both practitioners perform a complete assessment after they have centred and felt themselves to be in harmony with each other and the patient. Then the repatterning is carried out as if they were one unit, with the patient between them.

TO TOUCH OR NOT TO TOUCH?

As we have suggested, in learning about TT, there is no need to physically touch the patient (or even without the physical presence of the practitioner, when we look at the evidence for non-local healing). However, in practice most practitioners will use a combination of contact and non-contact TT in all its phases. Using touch appropriately at the right time and in the right place can help the practitioner stay centred and can bring an increased sense of wellbeing by the patient.

As indicated in Chapter 1, some westerners live in a particularly touch-deprived culture, and using gentle touch during a TT session can reinforce a sense of connection, that something is 'being done'. For many people, simple human contact is an added bonus on the journey towards healing. Practitioners will often include a good deal of hands-on contact in their TT work because patients often

Figure 4.9 *Two practitioners can work together.*

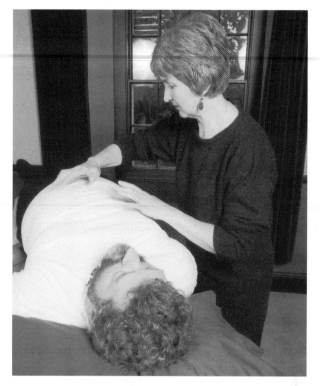

Figure 4.10 *Repatterning*

expect and are reassured by it. It can do no harm and may indeed enhance the patient's sense of wellbeing, and hence healing, when used judiciously and sincerely.

INTENTIONALITY

Other than centring, the most important quality necessary for TT to be a positive act for both of the people involved is intentionality. The practitioner must have a strong motivation to help or heal. Intentionality implies not only the will to help or heal but also a specific goal in mind, i.e. the practitioner understands how to facilitate the interaction. At the same time, it is necessary to give up the expectation of a particular change happening (see p. 115, compassionate non-attachment, for a further explanation).

The identification of intent is at least as important as the focus of the intent – perhaps more so. That is, in order to practice TT successfully, practitioners must acknowledge their motives. While intention to help patients achieve their maximum state of wellbeing is ideal, practitioners are also said to profit from trying to understand their desire to help.

In Rogers' (1970) model, intent is addressed under her concept of acausality. In this model everything and everyone – all energy fields – are interconnected. What each of us does directly affects everyone else. Therefore, the results of what one does are affected by other conditions, e.g. the other people involved, the environment in which it is done and so on. So it is possible to have intent to do something and yet for the effects to be quite different. The intent in playing billiards may be to shoot the ball, have it hit two others and have all three go into the pocket – but the results can be anywhere between that and none of them going in. The intent in turning a patient every hour may be to prevent pressure sores, but they may still occur. In spite of everything that has been discussed before, the intention of TT should not be to relieve symptoms, pain or anxiety but to creating 'wholeness' in the person. It is important to keep that intention of wholeness clear and then let go of desires for particular outcomes.

Inherent in this concept is the idea that by our thoughts, our focused consciousness, we influence the outcome of any interaction. One of the basic tenets of quantum physics is that we are not discovering reality, but participating in the creation of it.

We have often found that students of TT, naturally, want to relieve people's suffering or see an illness cured. This is a natural, if limited, human perspective, but it is important in TT to be aware that we cannot be sure of the meaning and purpose of suffering for another, or precisely what healing for another entails. It is better when working with patients, therefore, to pay particular attention to staying centred, to letting go of all our agendas, and simply to focus on being with the other in a loving and compassionate way as we bring all of our attention and intention upon them. Thus we can let go of ideas like, 'let the heart pain go away', such thoughts can be allowed to drift quietly into the background. It is better to simply hold an intention for the other, that they be healed, that they be whole – whatever that healing or wholeness might be for them.

COMPASSIONATE NON-ATTACHMENT

Practitioners sometimes have difficulty in understanding how one can have intentionality and yet be non-attached. They find it confusing to have an intention and yet let go of the outcome. The following case study addresses this confusion:

This experience was profound for me and I always think of it when I get personally attached to a certain outcome. No one can assume that they know what the outcome of TT will be. We can only visualise the patient whole and administer TT to them from a compassionate, non-attached place.

In the hospital in which I was working I was a primary nurse for a man I shall call Bill. Bill had lymphoma and had been a patient of mine for over a year – coming in for chemotherapy every few months. He had been a professor of physics at the university and was extremely interested in my experiences while learning TT. He always initiated a conversation around this subject whenever I cared for him, yet when I offered to do TT with him, he would always decline. However, his obvious interest in what I was doing, and indeed his confirmation of the things I was experiencing (from his physics background), was of great help to me. This was in the middle/late 1970s before I was aware of Rogers' framework.

One day I went to work and found Bill had been admitted and was in an acute and critical condition. As the shift wore on he became short of breath, his vital signs were not good and he developed a great deal of pain. While a decision was being made about his transfer to ICU, an X-ray was taken. He then said to me, 'you use TT to ease the dying, don't you?', to which I answered with a nod of my head. He then asked me to help him to die. On the assessment I felt a

Cont'd

blockage over the heart and intense, uneven energy in his forehead. I began to do TT with Bill, holding the intent in my mind of easing the transition for him. Thirty minutes later I felt his field to be balanced, but he was actually feeling much better and his vital signs were improving. I stayed with him for a while longer and then said goodbye as I had gone over my shift and was due back to work in just a few hours. However, neither one of us expected to see each other again. Coming back into work 8 hours later, I was met at the desk by a house officer who had in his hand two sets of X-rays – one that was taken prior to TT, one taken after I had left. The first X-ray showed evidence of a previous pulmonary embolus to his left lung, the second X-ray was clear of the embolus. No medical intervention had taken place. Bill had not been sent to ICU and he was looking much better. Ten days later, he died, but not before he had called to his bedside a sister from whom he'd been estranged for many years and with whom he was then reunited.

TT AND THE BENEFIT TO THE PRACTITIONER AND COLLEAGUES

Practitioners of TT may find themselves receiving immediate benefits from the relaxation and sense of wellbeing that comes from centring. In this state of consciousness, practitioners may experience unconditional love and compassion, which may have an added benefit by increasing the effectiveness of their immune system. If this is so, then this offers an explanation why practitioners of TT often report feeling better themselves after practising TT and seem to have less illness (Quinn 1993).

There may be other impacts arising from learning about TT among our colleagues and friends. As we remain more centred and focused, and deepen our own awareness of ourselves and our consciousness, then maybe others around us are influenced by this – family, friends, work colleagues. Learning about TT requires acceptance of considerable intimacy in our interactions and acceptance of others, it can therefore be of benefit if we want to strengthen our relationships among our teams at work, as the following vignette illustrates:

The enthusiasts for TT were easily persuaded to join the course. We set it up with them in mind. I was quite non-committal about TT myself, but was intrigued by its possibilities and prepared to give it a shot. We're just a small hospital here, yet people seem to work in their own little sectors and never seem to encounter each other, or work away behind the masks of their usual roles (not always for the best). Apart from watching staff beginning to use TT with patients (with some fascinatingly positive results) I was most impressed by the effect it has had on the staff. Twelve people participated in the introductory class, from a variety of different professions. Some of these used to be at each other's throats! The course transformed the way they work together. Their evaluations and my observations showed that something in the way they had to learn and practise TT brought new benefits, which I as a manager particularly appreciate. They report being more trusting of each other, less hooked-up on status, more focused on the patient as being at the centre of things. Some who were once near strangers or remote from each other behind professional boundaries, now greet each other as friends and work so much better together.

Director of hospital and community patient services.

'PROTECTION'

One of the questions most asked by students of TT is how to 'protect' themselves. When questioned what the protection is for they usually mention 'negative' or 'bad' energy from the patient, outside forces that might interfere with the process or take one over, and even 'evil spirits' or 'the Devil'.

Because the act of TT requires the practitioner to become sensitive and in tune with the other person (who is usually in some distress or imbalance), the practitioner may feel the mood, or the pain, of the patient if they are not centred. However, if we are able to maintain our own centre of consciousness, we recognise that this mood or pain is not our own. Although we may need to spend a moment in recentring, we quickly get back to the process itself – that of repatterning or rebalancing the patient's energy field into a synchronous flow. If we lose our intentionality and centre, and become identified with the patient and their problem, we will probably become part of the problem.

Practitioners find that moods are infectious. A joyous person quickly makes others happier. We 'pick up' sadness when we enter a room – or anger. Practitioners find that being in the presence of someone who is depressed can sap them of their energy very quickly. As we begin to be aware of the patterns and energy fields of others, and how the interaction of fields affects us, we recognise that the act of TT greatly intensifies projection, transference, countertransference, depression, anxieties (and likewise joy and feelings of wellbeing). We need to realise the importance of clear judgement about our own inner resources and ability to be of therapeutic value to others. Therefore centring is again of the utmost importance. When practitioners are calm and strong inside themselves, and can feel no personal investment in the outcome of the interaction, they are best able to set limits on how involved they want to become. Practitioners

---

ONE STUDENT'S SOLUTION TO TAKING ON THE PATIENT'S PROBLEMS

I had problems with tiredness and absorbing the client's excess energy during the first session. I could not believe her pain that I carried away with me. The weight and vice-like pain made me feel very muggy.

So I had to review my centring. Initially, I felt that I shouldn't have to keep centring myself during the treatment session but after my experience in the first session, in the second session, I stopped frequently to recentre. That was helpful but didn't cure it, so I tried another exercise that proved more effective.

However, I was still absorbing the patient's congestion to a lesser degree. I tried to shake the excess energy off my hands frequently and to wash my hands and have a drink of water after the session. But I felt the problem was in my method of using my hands in combination with my breathing. I was very sure that I was absorbing my patient's energy when I breathed in as I was working with her. So I tried to take both hands away whenever I breathed in, but this made the treatment disjointed and I often forgot to do it, in any case. I remembered my TT teacher saying how we give energy with out right and receive with our left. THE ANSWER! I changed my technique to closing my left hand whenever I breathed in during the treatment session. It worked! I am now giving TT without getting tired or absorbing congestion.

who are clear within themselves, centred and at the same time compassionate, with a deep intention to help or heal the whole patient, will not become adversely affected by the interaction (e.g. feel sapped of energy, experience pain in their own body or emotional distress). In other words, they will be 'protected'.

Sometimes, before the TT interaction, practitioners will include in the preparation an image of the interaction being surrounded by white light or some other similar image. If this makes the practitioner more secure then these exercises are encouraged. Those who still feel uncomfortable and in need of 'protection' after developing all of the above would probably do better practising another therapy.

> I have found that being very unattached to any outcomes for the patient is the best way I can take care of myself. In the past, after a TT session I would sometimes find myself feeling exhausted, nauseous or with a banging headache. I realised there was a pattern behind this on reflection, I wasn't taking care of myself by becoming too involved in what I hoped for the patient. It's all too easy when confronted with somebody's suffering to want to envisage their way out of it, to see them healed, free of pain, a painful problem resolved and so on. But I was sometimes so caught up in these desires I was depleted at the end of a session. Then I learned that by letting go of all this stuff, trusting to the right outcome to come up, a couple of interesting things happened. Firstly, I felt better. Secondly, the patients seemed to get more out of it too!
> TT practitioner

Although people have been using touch for many thousands of years as a means of helping and healing, we are only beginning to understand on a scientific basis our interconnectedness with all of life and what might be occurring in an energy field interaction, where the field is in the unified whole. However, everyone who is drawn to give TT would agree that they wish to do no harm. Even though harm can be done – usually on an emotional or spiritual level – by self-professed so-called 'healers' (see Chapter 1), the only uncomfortable side-effects reported by those who have received TT from practitioners properly trained by recognised TT organisations are (rarely) irritability, restlessness or sometimes an increase in anxiety. This sometimes manifests as actual pain felt by the patient in the area on which one is working, or as unexplained hostility coming from the patient. Krieger (1993) has noticed the same thing and calls it an 'energy overload'.

This can happen in beginners' classes when many people are exchanging experiences. An inexperienced healer who is trying too hard or someone who is trying to impress may also have this problem. It can also be observed when the practitioner begins the treatment from an overzealous state, which might arise from impulse, not intuition. In this case the practitioner is not acknowledging the intimate and emotional depth of the interaction nor being sensitive to the patients and their needs. Someone who is not centred can also cause discomfort to others. As in all energy interactions, the more sensitive the patient, the more care one must take.

Confidence is important in the act of TT. Confidence comes from knowing just how you are going to proceed and that you have the

> A good rule of thumb, I believe, is if you're unsure, don't. Do less rather than more. In TT you want to rebalance, repattern and modulate the patient's energy field into a synchronous flow, taking your cues from the assessment you make. No more, no less.
> TT practitioner

knowledge to deal with whatever may arise. This comes with practice and a continuously expanding knowledge base. TT looks very simple, and indeed it is. But what is really happening is hidden from view. TT is a paradox: although simple, it is one of the most complex of all interactions, and practitioners need to spend a lifetime working on themselves and gaining understanding of the concepts behind it.

Factors affecting success

TT is obviously not a therapy that all health care practitioners will choose to practice, nor is it the therapy of choice for all patients. Practitioners will get an intuitive sense of those who might respond, e.g. get a relaxation response and pain relief from TT. Occasionally this intuitive sense is wrong, but asking permission of the patient usually covers this. Asking for permission should be kept as simple as for instance, 'You seem a little tense', or 'it's not quite time for your pain medication. I've learned a technique that might help you. Would you like to try it?'. Students can create problems if they start trying to explain the theory behind TT or engage in a discussion of the new physics with their patient. All the patient usually wants is relief from discomfort, and discussion or explanation of the theory may or may not come later on in the relationship (informed consent and the legal aspects of TT will be discussed in Chapter 5).

After the practitioner has offered TT to a patient and they have agreed, there are other factors to consider which determine what kind of results will be achieved. These include the:

■ condition of the patient

■ patient's expectations

■ practitioner's degree of expertise.

CONDITION OF THE PATIENT

What is their diagnosis, prognosis? How long have they been in a state of imbalance or disease? What is their physical condition, emotional state, and spiritual awareness?

PATIENT'S EXPECTATIONS

Does the patient want to be different than they are? Do possible secondary gains through illness or pain outweigh the benefits of being different? For example, does the patient have some unwillingness to get well, perhaps because they do not wish to lose the regular visits by their nurse?

PRACTITIONER'S DEGREE OF EXPERTISE

Although almost anyone can learn the technique of TT in just a few minutes/hours and, with further teaching, confidence and practice the interaction will deepen and expand, it may take many years to become an expert practitioner. Some researchers have discounted studies where the practitioner had less than 3 years experience. This should not discourage practitioners – the best is yet to come! Even if we are still learning about our practice (and most TT practitioners would agree that we are always learning), our own learning journey is one of refinement and deepening of knowledge. As we have suggested, it is rare and difficult to harm others in TT along the way.

Joe was a young engineer who had been admitted to hospital because of a fungus infection. It had started between his toes, then spread to the top and bottom of his foot. His toes were swollen and there was a strong smell emitting from the raw, red areas. He also had a severe rash, due to the side-effects of the antibiotics, which spread from his groin to his stomach and a red itchy rash on his knees. He was barely able to walk and had calf-strain due to poor mobility.

After a simple explanation of TT, I stood at Joe's right hand side and centred on my breathing. I was aware of feeling very peaceful and sensitively aware of Joe's presence. I thought of him as being well and happy. I experienced a deepening sense of quiet, and lost awareness of all external noises and events. I felt purposeful and held the intent within me to help and heal. I felt deeply centred. I was now ready to assess Joe's energy field. Using long, sweeping, flowing movements from head to feet, my hands receptive to the cues I was receiving, I made a mental note of the areas where his field felt imbalanced. The left side of Joe's head and face felt hot, the neck felt difficult to pass my hands over. I felt pressure when I was in the area of the liver and the stomach. At the lower abdomen my hands felt a tingling sensation, which I also felt on his right foot and the last three toes of his left foot. When I assessed his back, I again had difficulty in passing my hands over the area of the liver, and a pulling sensation was felt in the middle of the back. The tingling over the right and left foot were the same. I cleared Joe's field using long sweeping movements of my hands. Continuing to feel my field interconnected with both Joe's field and the environmental field, I then projected, directed and modulated these energies until Joe sighed and looked relaxed. His breathing was also slower. I visualised the heat being dispersed from the side of Joe's face and head. I used short movements of my hands to change the energy imbalance, which I perceived as a dragging sensation, into one of harmony. My hands became very sensitive when working over the areas where I had sensed tingling. It was like receiving many tiny electrical impulses all across the palms of my hands. I continued modulating the energy field until Joe's field felt in balance.

Joe rested for 15 minutes and then he made comments such as, 'I'm sleepy and my foot feels great. It's quite extraordinary'. He later wrote on the diary sheet I had given him: 'During the treatment I felt warm sensations to various areas, which had been sore, itchy and watery. Near to the end of the treatment I could visualise, in my mind's eye, shimmering shapes which reminded me of net curtains being blown by a breeze in a darkened room. It felt as though objects were being placed on areas of my body during her treatment. After TT, I felt relaxed and contented.'

When I saw Joe for his second TT session, he reported that he was now experiencing no pain in his groin area and that he felt the rash 'had been responsive to TT treatment'. I followed the same phases as I had in the first. The left side of his head and face now felt balanced. His neck area was still slightly heavy and I modulated energy to disperse the congestion that I felt there. The groin area was considerably more even, but over the right foot my hands still felt a tingling sensation. I repatterned his whole energy field and, when I felt the field was more in harmony, I brought TT to an end.

In the third session, the only area where my hands felt an imbalance was in the lower abdomen and right foot. I used long sweeping movements over the lower abdomen, down the legs and onto the feet. This cleared the imbalance in the lower abdominal region. I then held my hands over his right foot for a few minutes visualising Joe as well and happy. I felt an increasing sense of peace and 'at-one-ness'. The feeling of unity with Joe deepened. It is hard to put into words the tranquil silence, where time seems to no longer exist. The quiescent moment of totality. As I passed my hands over the front of Joe once more, I felt that the TT session was completed. Joe began to snore. I sat by his side, still feeling an overwhelming calm.

THE PRACTITIONER'S WILLINGNESS AND ABILITY TO CONFRONT SELF AND MOTIVATION

The act of TT can look deceptively simple to an onlooker, it may look just like someone touching another person. In one of the research studies (Quinn 1982) 'mimic' TT was done as well as non-contact TT. Mimic TT is defined as an intervention that imitates the movements of the practitioner, but during which time there is no attempt to centre, no intention to assist the patient, no assessment of the condition of the patient and no conscious energy interaction. Both were recorded on video and the unpractised eye could not tell who was doing which. But the fact of the matter is that a great deal is happening inside the practitioner. Anyone can be shown how to make the hand movements associated with TT but, without centredness and the intention and motivation to help and heal, the results of TT are diminished or rendered ineffective. The practitioner's motivations in TT – whether to offer sincere help and healing to another or for some other benefit (e.g. acting out a need to have another dependent on them or need them, or for the sole purpose of making money) (Dass & Gorman 1986, Snow & Willard 1989, Wright & Sayre-Adams 2000) – will affect the degree of success of an episode of TT. People learn and apply TT for many different reasons, and part of the process of becoming an effective practitioner is to confront and examine motivations. Looking into the motivation for wanting to help will be a lifelong process, but it is necessary to make a start on this inner journey in order to become the kind of practitioner that professional practice demands. This exploration must be gentle and without guilt. It need not be shared with anyone, but it is sometimes helpful to share insights with a counsellor/supervisor or a trusted friend or colleague. Writing insights down in a journal can also be helpful. As more and more of us learn about TT, it will become easier to find colleagues to offer support and clinical supervision. Practitioners are far more likely to become and remain effective when they can seek guidance and help from others as well. Those who care for others need someone to care for them too.

REFERENCES

Dass R, Gorman P 1986 How can I help? Ryder, London
Krieger D 1979 The therapeutic touch: how to use your hands to help or heal. Prentice-Hall, Englewood Cliffs, New Jersey

Krieger D 1993 Accepting your power to heal. Bear & Co, Sante Fe

Krieger D, Ancoli S, Peper E 1979 Searching for evidence of physiological change. American Journal of Nursing 79(4):660–663

LeShan L 1974 How to meditate. Bantam, New York

Lionberger H 1985 An interpretive study of nurses' practice of therapeutic touch. Unpublished PhD dissertation, San Francisco, University of California.

Macrae J 1987 Therapeutic touch: a practical guide. Penguin, London

Peper E, Ancoli S 1976 Two endpoints of an EEG continuum of meditation. In: Krieger D (ed) 1979 Therapeutic Touch. Prentice Hall, London

Quinn J 1982 An investigation of the effects of therapeutic touch done without physical contact on the state of anxiety of hospitalised cardiovascular patients. Dissertation Abstracts International. University microfilm no. DA 82–26–7882

Quinn J 1993 Psychoimmunologic effects of therapeutic touch on practitioners and recently bereaved recipients: a pilot study. Advanced Nursing Science 15(4):13–26

Rogers M E 1970 An introduction to the theoretical basis of nursing. FA Davies, Philadelphia

Sayre-Adams J 1993 Therapeutic touch – principles and practice. Complementary Therapies in Medicine 1:96–99

Sayre-Adams J 1994 Therapeutic touch – a nursing function. Nursing Standard 8 (January 19):25–28

Snow C, Willard D 1989 I'm dying to take care of you. Professional Counsellor Books, Redmond, Washington

Wright S G, Sayre-Adams J 2000 Sacred space – right relationship and spirituality in healthcare. Churchill Livingstone, Edinburgh

5

Developing the practice

Jean Sayre-Adams   Steve Wright

The need for preparation
Consent and confidentiality
Deepening our understanding

■ *We shall not cease from exploration*
And the end of all our exploring
Will be to arrive where we started
And know the place for the first time.

T S ELIOT *Little Gidding*

Many health care workers have been caught up in the explosion of interest in complementary therapies in recent years. Some see this as a great opportunity to expand the boundaries of health care while others fear the uncontrolled application of these therapies (not to mention of the many 'unknowns' that surround them). All, including TT if we class it as a complementary therapy at this stage (but see the discussion in Chapter 1), have many potential benefits even though their mode of operation is often hard to define or substantiate in strictly rational or scientific terms.

The telephone message was from the senior staff nurse on one of the adult oncology wards, which use and support complementary therapies. The staff nurse is a qualified masseur, one of three who regularly treat the patients, but she had been unable to help the patient this time, and the physiotherapist would not attend without a doctor's referral. The message asked if there was anything that I could do to help urgently?

When I arrived, I asked the nurse for an update of the situation. It had begun as a simple movement of the head and a 'twinge', that ended in a spasm of torticollis. Now approximately 2 hours since the first movement, the patient was in 'excruciating pain and feeling helpless' as he curled further over the arm of his wheelchair in an effort to relieve it. I knelt in front of him, covered his clenched fists with my hands in greeting and looked into his pain-filled eyes. He was ashen, the fine diaphoresis covering his face and hands making his skin look even more transparent. The pain had rendered him helpless and vulnerable, he was unable to move, read, talk or swallow, and this meant not being able to take oral analgesics.

His scalp felt damp and cool on the surface, but by holding his head gently, heat could be felt, mostly on the right (twisted) side. Standing behind him, I placed my left hand on his forehead and gently and slowly massaged my right hand into the angle of his neck. As I held his head, I became aware of a deep, fine vibration in his neck. I asked him to breathe as slowly as possible and to allow the side of his neck to 'give' as it relaxed. I synchronised my breathing with his, allowing the energy to flow as we breathed out.

Cont'd

> Gradually, his neck relaxed and the tissues under my hand changed from tense and hot to softer and more even. With an audible sigh, his neck relaxed and he was able to look at me with a straight gaze. He smiled and said, 'I would never have believed it possible if I hadn't experienced it for myself'.
>
> Once back on his bed he was made comfortable and I completed the clearing that I felt was needed. As I continued from head to foot, I felt that the energy became more uniform in temperature and flow. Each time I returned to his head he would open his eyes and smile, following my hands with his gaze until his eyes closed and stayed closed as he surrendered into a restful, pain-free nap.

The need for preparation

When enthusiasm for a particular subject develops, one of the risks is the tendency to fall into 'quick fix' ways of learning about it. The proliferation of courses in complementary therapies extends from modules included in Masters Degree programmes and in-depth courses validated by reputable bodies to 'one-off' seminars and teaching sessions of dubious value, led by teachers with even more dubious qualifications. Unfortunately this plays into the hands of those who seek to vilify practitioners in complementary therapies as quacks and charlatans. Earlier chapters have suggested that there is a growing research and theoretical basis to support the practice of TT, and that it can be learned by anyone. It requires no special equipment and is not, at least in conventional terms, an invasive technique. However, the apparent simplicity of the practice of TT belies its fundamental complexity and intricacy. Thus, in Chapter 4 we have argued that no one should practise TT with patients unless they have satisfactorily completed a recognised programme of preparation as a practitioner.

Courses that teach TT are, however, only part of the commitment that we need to make. In Chapter 4, it was clearly identified that the success of TT depends not just on mastering the theory and practice, but also in the practitioner's continued development and exploration of themselves, their motives and purposes, what makes them 'tick', their spirituality, knowledge and expertise and so on. The chapter concluded that practitioners are best able to offer holistic help and healing to others when they are themselves learning about and developing themselves as well as their practice. Furthermore, they need to work in a culture that encourages and supports them in their skills (Wright & Sayre-Adams 2000).

The concept of clinical supervision, for example, is now strongly advocated for health care professionals (Butterworth & Faugier 1993). As the number of practitioners of TT expands, so too will the opportunity for them to seek clinical supervision by experts in their own field. The Sacred Space Foundation is currently offering support in this respect and strongly advocates that all TT practitioners should have access to a clinical supervisor with expertise in TT. The British Association of Therapeutic Touch (BATT) strongly advocates similar teaching and support.

Currently, the Sacred Space Foundation is the only body in the UK to offer a variety of accredited courses, from introductory 2-day seminars to longer programmes validated by professional bodies and universities. The course designed for practitioners lasts a year and includes formal teaching sessions, the use of reflective practice, clinical supervision, case study and dissertation work.

REPORTS FROM STUDENTS OF TT CLASSES

'The energy literally sizzled in the space between my hands and his palms. It is all so special and yet so ordinary.'

'At a time when before I have felt rather helpless and would possibly have avoided the patient, I now feel that there is something to offer, not only to the patient, but it may also offer comfort to the relatives. By showing them the basic TT techniques, it gives them a means to communicate and it may be that this helps in the commencement of the grieving process.'

'There is the personal pleasure of having learnt a new skill, plus the stimulation and excitement that comes with satisfaction as new knowledge is acquired. The information gained from being able to offer a new concept can only bring benefit to existing nursing practices.'

REPORTS FROM STUDENTS OF TT CLASSES *Cont'd*

'Like a bird on the wing has an expanded vision, so Therapeutic Touch has expanded my horizon.'

'My whole horizon has been opened up by the experience of TT. This in turn has been reflected in my work, both in my written work and my practical work and also of course in everything I do. It's almost like being a new person, certainly a wiser one.'

'I am more grounded than I used to be.'

'The deeper I enter this awakening within, the more difficult it becomes for me to express it in words. I feel as if I have found myself.'

'Without emotional attachment but with a loving care I can see my weaknesses and strengths, and this is helping me to grow, because I can accept me as I am. Knowing that I am not perfect, and that this is part of me, helps me to reach others because I too have lumps and bumps and cracks and wrinkles that are part of me, and makes the wholeness real. Before, I had great difficulty in acknowledging these parts. They were too painful, too hateful, too mortifying. Now they are the light and dark that an artist has used to get the effect of depth and realness.'

'One of the most rewarding aspects of my work is to show parents ways of coping with the stresses of family life. There is often that feeling of helplessness when caring for a crying, fretful or sick child, which soon can lead to loss of confidence in themselves as parents. By teaching the simple technique of TT to parents, they then feel they have something special to offer, which in time increases their self-esteem and so strengthens the bond between them and their child.'

Students undertaking a TT course frequently find it to be a transformative experience. The sense of learning and excitement in their evaluations is almost palpable.

The personal development and pleasure that students may get from a TT course, however worthy in themselves, are not sufficient to substantiate it in practice. Practitioners need to be safe, not only to maintain the credibility of a particular therapy but, most importantly, to maintain public safety and confidence.

Many professional organisations require practitioners to demonstrate competence in any technique they use in their practice. In the case of nursing, for example, the Code of Professional Conduct (UKCC 1992a) is very explicit about the goals of nurses to, 'act, at all times, in such a manner as to safeguard and promote the interests of individual patients and clients'. Each nurse is 'personally accountable' for his or her practice, and may be subject to disciplinary action, even removal from the register of nurses (meaning that he or she will no longer be able to practice as such). BATT and other complementary therapy organisations have adopted similar strict codes of conduct.

Thus nurses are required to demonstrate that their professional knowledge and practice is up to date. When they add new dimensions to their practice (such as learning about working as a practitioner of TT) they must do so only if they can demonstrate adequate preparation that makes them competent to offer such a service. Indeed, organisations such as the Royal College of Nursing (RCN), which includes indemnity insurance in its membership fees, make the same requirement of their members if they are to maintain their insurance cover. Fortunately, litigation by dissatisfied patients against nurses and other practitioners is still relatively rare, and it is important to keep the risks in proportion. People who feel cared for very seldom resort to litigation. However, when nurses ask whether they are 'covered' to give TT, one of the factors that govern the response is whether or not the person offering it can demonstrate competence through properly validated training. One of the common concerns registered by critics of complementary therapies is the lack of controls over who can practise them. In the UK, wider Europe and the United States, for example, there is wide variation in standards of training and professional control. Legislation and professional accountability are invariably later developments to a new healing approach.

Where practitioners are governed by professional codes of conduct, this at least appears to offer the public protection. Professional bodies (such as the United Kingdom Central Council; UKCC) have recognised that nurses, for example, must expand their practice in many ways beyond initial graduation and registration, and have reinforced the personal accountability of nurses when they do so (UKCC 1992b). The UKCC has recognised that expecting nurses to hold a 'certificate' for every additional practice they undertake may be overly simplistic. Instead, it has emphasised adherence to a number of 'principles of practice', including the need to maintain and develop knowledge and competence underpinning any aspect of nursing practice in order to promote patient safety.

Consent and confidentiality

The maintenance of patient confidentiality and consent to treatment with TT is governed by the same principles applicable to any health care intervention.

A 23-year-old woman with whom I work was in the beginnings of a migraine. I offered to do some TT with her. As she agreed she told me she was uptight about her situation and wanted help to relax and perhaps some feedback as to how she could take responsibility to make changes in her life that would help her avoid getting in the state in which her migraines occurred.

I began treatment with the patient lying supine on the bed – she did not want to turn over, but preferred to remain on her back throughout the treatment. I carefully supported her arms and the area underneath her knees with pillows to allow her position to facilitate maximum relaxation.

I began by explaining how we affect one another's energy fields and that I may work with my hands in contact with her body sometimes and at other times hold my hands a little way from her body. I told her that her discomfort was likely to start to subside and continue to do so after treatment if it was not completely gone at the end of the session. I also asked her to raise her right hand if she wanted me to stop the treatment for whatever reason, and then tell me what her needs were in her own time. I told her that she could help with her treatment by picturing a 'letting go' of her discomfort and seeing herself in full health. I prepared her to expect to lie quiet for 20–30 minutes after the session.

During the centring I stood at the head end of the patient with the top of her head facing me and stayed this way for about 5 minutes. She gradually relaxed, her facial expression became softer and her breathing deepened and slowed.

If I start 'thinking' and 'planning' what I am to do, beyond holding the general framework in the background of my mind, I become self-conscious and end up doing something *to* the patient and get attached to the results. The 'centring' process is about tuning in to the 'intuition' and letting whatever comes flow. When my 'self' gets out of the way there is a deep inner 'knowing' that I touch, a process on a deeper level. Words are very clumsy tools for expressing this process.

When she seemed really relaxed, I did the assessment on her.

I felt areas of congestion, heaviness and blockages. There were some cooler areas as well as emotional tension and conflict.

I had a sense of the left side absorbing energy, the right side felt stagnant. I worked in an anticlockwise circular movement until the energy was flowing more and more freely. Next I worked with my hands about 4–6 inches away from the body and 'smoothed' the whole energy field from head to toe. The main part of the treatment involved holding my right hand fairly close to the left side of the throat area and the left hand fairly close to the face and crown. I had a picture of blue–white light flowing from my left hand and being directed by my right hand. After about 5 minutes I 'knew' it was time to stop and I completed the session with a quick check of the general energy field and balance of the feet. Some tears appeared while I held my hands near the neck area – there was a sense of something being released. The patient was almost asleep at the end of the session and I woke her up after half an hour's rest. She felt ready to get up and go.

Consent to any treatment may be 'implied', for example, the patient in the hospital bed or attending a private therapy session is presumed to have submitted him/herself to a reasonable range of care. Thus, every time a practitioner pursues a particular activity with a patient, it is not necessary for a consent form to be signed. However, it is still open to debate as to how far TT can yet be considered part of mainstream health care. In some settings, it may be necessary for patients, or their guardians, to be asked to sign consent forms when TT is offered, although this tends to be unusual. Experience suggests that most nurses and other health care workers are learning to offer TT as part of their normal range of helping and healing activities.

A more critical factor is the need for consent to be informed. As the above example illustrates, explaining what TT is all about to the patient beforehand is important, giving the patient an opportunity to ask questions and give or deny permission. Such explanations need to be in terms that the patient understands, and they should give realistic expectations of the effects.

An increasing emphasis is being placed on health care professionals working in 'partnership' with patients and clients. This trend away from the authoritarian ('I know best') professional and the passive ('I'm in your hands') appears to be a universal phenomenon, reinforced by government policies in many countries, such as the Patient's Charters in the UK, which place greater emphasis on patients' rights and empowerment in health care delivery. Of course, patients' responses to health care workers can be extremely variable. Some patients may wish the professionals to 'take control' while others will demand information and control over all elements of their care. It is important to be able to respond to all the different approaches along this continuum.

Empowering patients and clients by giving information is a significant feature. They are better able to be involved in the decision-making process and give informed consent if they know what is on offer, and if they have confidence in the practitioner. Some organisations have risen to this challenge, such as the Complementary Therapies Forum at the Royal College of Nursing in the UK, which has produced guidance for users of complementary therapies to help them get the information they need. It suggests (RCN 1993) a number of questions, which the user should ask before accepting treatment from a practitioner:

- What are the practitioner's qualifications and how long was their training?

- Are they a member of a recognised, registered body, with codes of practice?

- Can they give you the address and telephone number of this to check?

- Is the therapy available on the NHS?

- Can the patient's GP delegate their care to the practitioner?

- Is this the most appropriate complementary therapy for the patient's problem?

- Will the practitioner send a letter to the patient's GP advising him/her of any treatment received?

- Can the patient claim for the therapy through their private health insurance scheme, if they have one?

- Are the practitioner's records confidential?

- What is the cost of the treatment?

- How many treatments should the patient expect to need (and therefore approximate cost)?

- What insurance cover does the practitioner have?

Mr W came to the clinic suffering with a pain in his right foot, which had been troubling him for some 18 months, and also with a pain in his right shoulder and neck, which had been present for a few months. The injury to Mr W's foot had occurred while on holiday. He had dived into a swimming pool and on doing so felt 'something go' in his heel and thereafter had suffered pain and stiffness in this area. This discomfort varied in intensity depending on how much walking he did and the type of shoe worn. The pain in his neck and shoulder had no explicable cause. Mr W is 57 years old and works as a clerk in a local public transport services department.

On Mr W's first visit, he looked very apprehensive as he did not know what TT entailed. I reassured him by explaining that all that was required of him was to remove his shoes, lie on the couch and make himself comfortable. I further explained that I would simply pass my hands over his body in order to assess and rebalance his energy field, which I explained in simple terms. Mr W seemed satisfied with this explanation, and asked no more questions.

Cont'd

After Mr W had made himself comfortable on the couch, I proceeded to centre myself by visualising an oak tree with its leaves shimmering in the gentle breeze and inwardly calming myself by taking a few deep breaths, focusing on the intention to help and heal.

Following this I carried out an initial assessment of Mr W's energy field by placing my hands parallel to each other, a few inches above his body surface and, starting from the head, moved my hands down towards his feet, in a continuous flowing motion. Mr W had a distinct coolness over his right foot, which indicated a blocked area of tight congestion. When asked if this was the foot troubling him, he confirmed that this was so.

As this blockage was present, I placed my hands under the arches of Mr W's feet and directed energy into this area to penetrate and loosen the congestion. This I did for a couple of minutes. This was enough for the blockage to move and energy to flow evenly in both feet.

I then reassessed the energy field but did not pick up any new cues, although the foot still felt cool. Therefore, I continued to energize the foot in order to promote the circulation of the energy flow. When the area began to feel warm, I discontinued this approach and carried out further reassessment and rebalancing of the whole energy field.

Following this, I then carried out an assessment of Mr W's back, from head to feet. Again I felt coolness around the neck and shoulder, and energised this area and thereafter reassessed and rebalanced the whole energy field.

The treatment lasted for approximately 20 minutes and when I had finished, Mr W asked 'Is that it?' Mr W had not felt any sensations, for example warmth or tingling, and obviously wondered what it was all about. I explained that not everyone experienced sensations but that did not mean no beneficial effect would be experienced.

While I carried out the treatment, I remained centred, focusing my attention on helping Mr W to be well and balanced. When rebalancing the whole field, I visualised warm light spreading throughout the body.

Although Mr W did not seem convinced that anything had been done to help him, he did make a further appointment for the following week.

When he arrived the following week, he informed me that almost as soon as he had left the clinic the previous week, the pain in his right foot had much improved and for most of that intervening week, he had been pain-free, although the pain in his neck and shoulder remained.

On that second visit, I carried out the treatment as for the previous week, energising the foot and shoulder areas in order to relieve congestion gathered there and drawing it out through the extremities and giving an overall rebalancing. On this occasion Mr W did experience a warm sensation in his foot.

The third treatment was carried out as for the previous weeks but on assessment, the foot area definitely did not feel cool as it had on the first, and Mr W was very pleased in the improvement, as he said that some days previous to treatment he had been unable to walk downstairs due to the pain. As the shoulder and neck remained painful, I spent more time on this area, directing energy to loosen the congestion as coolness was still felt in this area. I visualised a warm, light stream of energy penetrating a knot and slowly undoing it.

On the fourth and final visit, Mr W said he felt a fraud coming, as he felt so much better, the pain in his foot, neck and shoulder having been relieved. Even though he felt better I carried out an assessment of his energy field and it felt more complete with no cool areas being detected. The treatment was completed with an overall rebalancing of the energy field.

Unknown to me, Mr W suffers with arthritis in his left hip, which causes him pain and is now more tolerable having received TT.

Asking such questions will help to ensure that participation in TT is based on informed consent, and also reduce the risk of exposure to bad practice. Members of the public who are unsure about what is the best service on offer can be encouraged to consider questions such as these and elicit satisfactory responses before putting themselves in the hands of a practitioner.

Deepening our understanding

There are great shifts occurring in all of our ways of thinking and doing things as the new millennium begins. Sometimes the changes seem too fast and too radical for the individual to feel comfortable with. However, many believe that we can replace the systems that no longer serve us and participate in creating environments that will support healing. In the preceding chapters, we have looked at the history of healing, of laying on of hands and of Therapeutic Touch (TT). We have seen the attitude of society to this healing art and, as the contemporary shift occurs, it is clear that TT is slowly gaining not only acceptance but also popularity.

Health care professionals are flocking to the healing arts because they long to put the heart back into our health care systems. They are interested in TT because they see it brings relaxation, healing and pain relief to their patients. There is beginning to be an aware-ness of the conceptual framework that is often used for TT, which satisfies the need to know why. Since research was first begun on TT in 1975, we have seen large amounts of research coming particularly from North America by nurses in their masters' and doctors' degrees.

The need for more research is evident, and is reinforced by Quinn (1992):

> *The first and perhaps most obvious (need) is the application of TT to a host of real world clinical problems – clinical trials or outcome studies. The second path involves the development of an explanatory model/theory of TT that is validated and refined through the research process.*

A deepening of understanding around Rogers' field theory, and perhaps other theories that might more appropriately explain how TT works (see Chapter 1), as well as continued and replicated studies on TT, is needed. However, the evidence shows that interest in and commitment of TT has grown rapidly among practitioners for essen-tially one reason – it seems to work (Sayre-Adams 1993). TT offers an important dimension in healing and caring for many health care professionals. Research so far suggests that it can bring significant benefits to patients, at minimal cost. At the same time, no harmful effects have yet been demonstrated when TT is done by practitioners who have been trained by Krieger or her students and follow the guidelines set up by the governing bodies of TT.

The challenges that are being presented in many different countries to professional bodies mirror the challenges in North America.

Professional nursing bodies such as the American Holistic Nurses Association and the Nurse Healers Professional Association, as well as The Therapeutic Touch Network in Canada, are also talking about regulation and educational standards for those who practice TT. The British Association of Therapeutic Touch is likewise struggling with these challenges.

There are two ways of looking at or conceptualising the place of practitioners in the health care environment. One is to see the carer and the patient as innocent victims of a decaying, worn out, ineffective system. The other is to see the health care professional and the patient as conscious participants in the changing of the system. Barrett (1990) says:

> *Nursing care in this [Roger's] system is concerned with patterning the environmental field. The nurse, together with the client, patterns the environment to promote healing and comfort.*

If, regardless of professional background, we chose to look at our health care system from this second view, the kinds of questions that arise are, 'What can we do to create a healing environment for the patient?' 'How can the environment be changed?' When we turn our attention to these questions, the issues of colour, light, sound, activity, temperature take on importance. 'Regardless of the practice modality being used, the nurse's objective is to pattern the client's environment to promote health and well being' (Barrett 1990). Barrett and others have focused on nursing, but the potential is enormous for large numbers of others within the health care system to begin to alter the environment by the use of lighting, imagery, relaxation, music therapy and art therapy. They can promote the health and wellbeing of their patients by the use of massage, aromatherapy and TT, as well as other complementary therapies.

However, considering the conceptual framework that incorporates the theoretical perspectives suggested by Rogers (1970, 1986, 1990), expanded by Newman (1979, 1982, 1986, 1990) and tested by Quinn (1984, 1989b, 1992) and others, what of the idea that the health care practitioner may become the environment of the patient? Quinn (1992) writes:

In this perspective, the nurse turns toward his or her understanding of the 'nurse' as an energetic, vibrational field, integral with the patient's environment. When the focus is on the nurse as the environment the questions that arise are 'How can I be a more healing environment? How can I use my consciousness, my being, my voice, my touch, my face, for healing?' What are the limits of influence if the means of influence is an energy field?

It is necessary to review the conceptual framework that Rogers introduced into nursing in 1970. This conceives the fundamental unit of the living system as an energy field, coextensive with the environmental energy field. Although at the time, this was a revolutionary idea in health care, and an unacceptable conjecture of little or no interest to Western medicine, a quarter of a century later, one cannot approach the cutting edge of practically any modern scientific discipline, nor the tradition of any major spiritual culture, and not see the same idea proposed. No longer merely conjecture, the interconnectedness of all life seems clear. Scholars, artists, and futurists alike are writing about this phenomenon in fields as diverse and different from each other as quantum physics, biology, psychology, psychoneuro-immunology, philosophy, theology, spirituality and medicine. We find it being expressed too in painting, music, poetry, prose and dance. The emerging view of our world includes the concepts that the human being is a non-material, multi-dimensional field integral with the environment/universal field; that consciousness is non-local, unbounded by physical structure and function; and that the separateness of the individual from all other life forms is a reductionist and limited view.

HEALING ENVIRONMENTS

Taking these basic assumptions, we need to explore the potential of this model of reality for creating healing environments. A healing environment is one that facilitates the emergence of the multi-dimensional response of people in the direction of healing and wholeness. Quinn (1992) wrote:

Healing, the emergence of right relationship at, between, and among all the levels of human being, is always accomplished by the one healing. No-one and nothing can heal another human being. All healing is creative emergence, new birth, the manifestation of the powerful inner longing, at every level, to be whole.

What, then, is the role for the health care worker? Nightingale (1869) believed nurses could remove barriers to the healing process:

The role of the nurse is to put the patient in the best possible position for nature to act.

Quinn (1992) believes the same:

The nurse can participate in creating environments that will support healing. The nurse can become a midwife to the process of healing, creating and being safe. The nurse can be the sacred space into which the healing might emerge. The nurse can, literally, BECOME the healing environment.

Further, taking from these theorists and disciplines the basic assumption that we are interconnected to all life, our consciousness is not separate and apart but integral with all consciousness. Nor is such a view restricted to the nursing examples we have given here (although, in relation to TT, it seems that it is nurses who have taken the lead). The health care professional can become a conscious participant in the web of interconnectedness towards repatterning and healing for ourselves and for others through the intentional use of our own consciousness. The clinical practice of TT is an example of this participation: the first and most important step in TT is a shift in the consciousness of the practitioner (in the act of centring). Through this, clinical experience and empirical study demonstrate, there can also be a shift in consciousness of the recipient. Cowling (1990) writes that the practitioner:

...could knowingly participate in human field patterning through his/her interconnectedness to the client, possible in a four-dimensional [pan-dimensional] universe of open fields. For instance, it has been suggested that a human-to-human field process operates in TT through the mode of ... intentionality on the part of the practitioner.

Intentionality is an important concept in the practice of TT.

TUNING IN

Quinn (1992) writes:

What may actually be happening in the act of TT is that the practitioner, through the act of centring, is repatterning his/her own energy field in the direction of expanded consciousness, a consciousness experienced as unified, harmonious, peaceful, ordered, and understood to be a 'healing meditation'. It is proposed that being in the TT process with a practitioner in such an expanded (meditative) state of consciousness may provide a template of sorts upon which the patient may repattern.

Using the metaphor of sound, the pattern of vibration of the practitioner's consciousness, 'becomes a tuning fork, resonating at a healing frequency, and the patient has the opportunity within the mutual person–environment process to attune, to resonate, to that frequency'. (Quinn 1992).

This perspective, along with the 'timelessness' that TT practitioners experience (explored by Newman 1982, 1990 and Quinn 1993) inclines us to shift from previous (pre-1993) descriptions of the basis behind TT, which utilise an 'energy exchange' model that includes a here and a there – a source and a recipient of energy – to a model of interconnectedness (to which this text inclines), in which there is no here or there, there is just now – and always.

The poet T S Eliot put it another way in *East Coker* (from *Four Quartets*):

In order to arrive at what you are not
  You must go through the way in which you are not.
And what you do not know is the only thing you know
And what you own is what you do not own
And where you are is where you are not.

There is a challenge for all health care professionals who aspire to practice holistically, i.e. who accept the basic premise of holism, of an interconnected universe, and of the fundamental inseparability of individuals one from the other to move out of the 'victim' role so often adopted and begin to be conscious participants in the creation of healing environments. In this view the systems are not some alien, separate being with a life of their own, but part of us. *We* are the environment. We are the systems we work in. By changing and expanding our consciousness, we can become the facilitators for change – first in ourselves, then perhaps our patients, our systems, our planet.

Stories abound of the potential for change when a critical mass of people change their consciousness and decide that things have to change (see for example Watson's (1980) much-quoted '100th monkey' phenomenon, or the assumptions of transcendental meditation that social change can occur when enough people meditate in a particular way (Quinn 1992)). These optimistic stories suggest that we can indeed make the world into a different place when enough of us want it to be so. Anyone who watched the Berlin Wall come down would find some strength in this argument.

Whether this phenomenon is true or not is open to question. What does seem possible is that the many walls that exist in the world of health care are vulnerable to demolition if enough of us decide that the limitations we currently experience no longer serve us or our patients or clients. A commitment to TT invites us to tear down the many walls within and between us and venture into new reality, rich with the potential to bring healing for all.

REFERENCES

Barrett E A M 1990 Health patterning with clients in a private practice environment. In: Barrett E A M (Ed) Visions of Rogers' science-based nursing. National League for Nursing, New York

Butterworth A, Faugier J 1993 Clinical supervision and mentorship in nursing. Chapman & Hall, London

Cowling W R 1990 A template for unitary pattern-based nursing practice. In: Barrett E A M (Ed) Visions of Rogers' science-based nursing. National League for Nursing, New York

Newman M 1979 Theory and development in nursing. F A Davies, Philadelphia

Newman M 1982 Time as an index of expanding consciousness with age. Nursing Research 31(5):290–293

Newman M 1986 Health as expanding consciousness. Mosby, St Louis

Newman M 1990 Newman's theory of health as praxis. Nursing Science Quarterly 3(1):37–41

Nightingale F 1869 (1980 edn.) Notes on nursing – what is, what it is not. Churchill Livingstone, Edinburgh

Quinn J 1984 Therapeutic Touch as energy exchange: testing the theory. Advances in Nursing Science 6(2):42–49

Quinn J 1989a Future directions for Therapeutic Touch research. Journal of Holistic Nursing 7(1):19–25

Quinn J 1989b Therapeutic Touch as energy exchange: replication and extension. Nursing Science Quarterly 2(2):79–87

Quinn J 1992 Holding sacred space: the nurse as healing environment. Holistic Nursing Practice 6(4):26–36

Quinn J 1993 Psychoimmunologic effects of Therapeutic Touch on practitioners and recently bereaved recipients: a pilot study. Advances in Nursing Science 15(4):13–26

RCN (1993) Complementary therapies – a consumer checklist. RCN, London

Rogers M E 1970 An introduction to the theoretical basis for nursing. F A Davies, Philadelphia

Rogers M E 1986 Science of unitary human beings. In: Malinski V M (ed) Explorations on Martha Rogers' science of unitary human beings. Appleton-Century-Crofts, Norwalk, Connecticut

Rogers M E 1990 Nursing: science of unitary, irreducible, human beings: update (1990). In: Barrett E A M (ed) Visions of Rogers' science-based nursing. National League for Nursing, New York

Sayre-Adams J 1993 Therapeutic Touch. In: Trevelyan J, Booth B (eds) Complementary therapy. Nursing Times Sourcebook, London

UKCC 1992a The code of professional conduct. The United Kingdom Central Council for Nursing, Midwifery and Health Visiting, London

UKCC 1992b The scope of professional practice. The United Kingdom Central Council for Nursing, Midwifery and Health Visiting, London

Watson L 1980 Lifetide. London, Bantam

Wright S G, Sayre-Adams J 2000 Sacred space – right relationship and spirituality in healthcare. Churchill Livingstone. Edinburgh

6
Conclusions

Jean Sayre-Adams   Steve Wright

■ *The day will come when,*
after harnessing the winds, the tides,
and gravity, we shall harness for God
the energies of love. And on that day,
for the second time in the history of
the world, man will have discovered fire.

TEILHARD DE CHARDIN

So far we have sought to identify the research and theoretical basis for TT, and the central issues in its practical application. A number of key points are worth summarising:

- TT is a harmless technique that promotes a balanced state, aiding those involved to enter the best possible position for relaxation and maximum health to occur.

- TT is an innate approach to human caring that can be learned by anyone who so desires.

- There is a need to carry out more research into TT, including rigorous identification of patient outcomes as health care systems worldwide focus more and more on 'cost-effectiveness', 'evidence-based medicine' and 'value for money

- As more and more health care professionals and others learn about and practice TT, they will be able to contribute to expanding its theoretical underpinnings. At the same time there is an opportunity to draw upon relevant and related concepts from many other fields of thinking.

- Education for the practice of TT needs to be well validated, using a wide range of enlightened techniques. The Sacred Space Foundation in the UK and the Nurse Healers Professional Association (NHPA) in the United States, for example, are already advanced in this field. Standards of education and practice should conform to the requirements of the reputable bodies that regulate practitioners and their training.

- All practitioners must undertake recognised programmes, be registered with their own professional body and have appropriate insurance cover. The protection of patients is paramount.

- Practitioners need continuous updating and access to clinical supervision. Where they work in health care organisations, then a supportive culture and climate is needed, which is conducive to health and the support of both practitioner and patient.

- TT does not stop with the practitioner–patient relationship. Its significance has ramifications into the work of all carers, the health care system and society as a whole.

As interest in TT expands, it is important to examine it not just from the perspective of a new technique to be added to the existing practices of nurses and other health care workers, or to see it as just another therapy. Nor, as we have tried to suggest in these pages, is TT a simple linear relationship from healer to patient. There is a grander perspective to view – that of engaging in the intricate and dynamic dance of the cosmos. The potential, when thousands of health care professionals and others participate intentionally in this dance, is to transform the health and wellbeing of millions of people. TT is not a panacea; it will not cure every patient nor will it cure all the health system's ills or help all patients love all their carers all of the time. It is, however, part of what may be seen as a worldwide movement for change. It changes those who participate in it, and they in turn may participate in changing the world. It is a piece of the jigsaw puzzle in the search for health that, when locked into place, helps us to appreciate the bigger picture – the awesome picture – in which we find ourselves.

All things in heaven come about in existence
Existence comes about in non-existence …
Both are one in origin
and different only in name.
Its unity is called the secret.
The secret's still deeper secret
is the gateway through which all miracles
emerge.

Tao Te Ching

USEFUL ADDRESSES

British Association of Therapeutic Touch (BATT), Ravenscroft, Renwick, Cumbria CA10 1JL, UK
Nurse Healers Professional Association (NHPA), 3760 South Highland Drive, Salt Lake City, Utah 84106, USA
Sacred Space Foundation, Redmire, Mungrisdale, Cumbria CA10 0TB, UK
The Therapeutic Touch Network, 4009 Bloor Street West, Toronto, ON M9B 1M4, Canada

Index

Page numbers in **bold** type refer to illustrations and tables.